Writing the Wisdom

*Creative writing as response
to childhood trauma*

— BARBARA GLASSON —

— PENNY JOHNSON —

Sacristy
Press

Sacristy Press
PO Box 612, Durham, DH1 9HT

www.sacristy.co.uk

First published in 2022 by Sacristy Press, Durham

Sacristy Limited, registered in England
& Wales, number 7565667

British Library Cataloguing-in-Publication Data
A catalogue record for the book is
available from the British Library

ISBN 978-1-78959-207-8

Contents

Contents

Introduction

This is a story of exploration and discovery, a story of friendship and attentiveness to shocking experiences and profoundly courageous human beings. It is a challenging story; it challenges both individuals and communities to listen differently. It is a story of human resilience in the face of fragmentation and trauma. It is a story about what might be possible for those in pastoral ministry. It is a story about the transformation of lives and institutions. It is a small story of collaboration between a pastor and a counsellor. It is a story about human wisdom and the power of words. It is an unfinished story.

Who are we?

The overlap between pastoral care and counselling can be a difficult one. The pastor, after all, is trained in what has been quaintly described as "the cure of souls", a discipline that involves being alongside others which is both prayerful and spiritual. Whilst the counsellor also shares this desire to accompany, the issues of spirituality and faith can be viewed as outside the discipline of enabling another to express their unique experiences and identity. There can be suspicion in this relationship, the pastor seeing the counsellor as a remote professional, whilst the counsellor can view the pastor as someone with an unhelpful agenda of spiritual baggage. Those who describe themselves as "Christian counsellors" might be viewed with suspicion on both sides, neither boundaried professionals nor wise priests, wanting to impart their own views to vulnerable people via the medium of counselling. So, in the middle of these stereotypes, we can say from the outset that this journey was unusual: a partnership between a Methodist minister and a counsellor who happens to be a Christian, that partnership and the overlap between the two disciplines being discovered through the imaginative medium of words.

What brought us together?

The reason for the overlap was that both the counsellor, Penny, and the pastor, Barbara, had found themselves alongside others who variously described themselves as "survivors" or "victims" or "freedom fighters"—people who had experienced the trauma of abuse in their early life and whose adult years had become disrupted and fragmented by memories of these experiences. Some of these memories had not yet emerged as a coherent story but were expressed through the relived trauma of flashbacks, dissociation, memory loss or spiritual, physical or emotional distress. This had presented to both Penny and Barbara in ways that were fragmented and challenging; they both felt themselves called to listen and learn, to hold fast to the process of accompaniment and to try, in whatever way they could, to stay faithful to the accounts of trauma they were both hearing.

At the point of meeting, both Barbara and Penny were working at Holy Rood House in Thirsk, a centre for health and healing in North Yorkshire. Penny had a number of clients coming to her on a regular basis for therapy. Barbara was working as a Methodist minister in Liverpool City Centre where she had encountered a number of people who were telling her their stories of abuse and its resultant trauma. She had been working alongside these people in ways that felt far beyond her theological training, and she was taking time at Holy Rood House to try to assess and reflect on what makes for sound pastoral practice.

What did we do and why?

The conversations between Penny and Barbara began in Thirsk, and a mutual respect for the two disciplines of counselling and pastoral care became a topic for shared exploration. In this dialogue, it became apparent that there was the possibility of working together to create a safer space for people who had experienced abuse to tell their stories differently. To this end, Barbara and Penny initiated and led a few residential retreats entitled "Women Breaking Free" in which small groups of women were invited to spend time together, exploring their experiences through creative means, sharing self-help strategies, eating around the same table and being together in supportive ways. A key part to these weekends was an exploration of creative writing.

In the Women Breaking Free weekends a number of discoveries were made. Firstly, the sheer bravery of women who had suffered significant trauma in signing up for such an unknown event was astonishing. Even to fill out the application form was an immense test of courage as it meant that the participant was "out" as a survivor in ways that many had not previously experienced. This was apparent in the nervousness of the correspondence that happened in advance of the weekend and in the palpable anxiety as people came to the door and rang the bell. Some women came in secret as their families did not know of their previous experiences; others were struggling with the fragmentation of their divided, dissociated selves. Throughout the weekend, the women began to relax and to share, both through conversations in the group and in one-to-one conversations with Barbara and Penny. This needed very clear boundaries; there was no secret that Barbara was an ordained minister, whilst Penny was clear that the conversations were not part of any formal counselling agreement. For some, talking to an ordained person was helpful; for others it was to be avoided at all costs! There was no overt religious symbolism on show, neither were any counselling notes taken.

The weekends were challenging and at times difficult, where it was necessary to prepare and enable participants to share appropriately and to be able to return home safely. Although there were moments of deep distress as memories were expressed, there was also much laughter, mutual support and creativity. In particular, through some prompts and encouragement, the women began to write the most extraordinary and moving stories and poems, which, with permissions, Penny collected into an anthology.

The Women Breaking Free weekends became popular and, having experienced one, the same women wanted to come again and again. However, the financial cost of a residential weekend and the emotional cost to those running it were considerable, and the work paused for a while to consider next steps.

Subsequently, Barbara went to work in the city centre of Bradford at a Methodist project called Touchstone and Penny came through to the Touchstone centre each week to meet a number of clients. It was no longer possible to have residential weekends, but the opportunity of gathering people together to develop the creative writing process continued to feel important. As a result, a number of day retreats were organized and different shapes and sorts of poems were attempted.

Why are we sharing this with you?

Penny and Barbara's work together has grown out of increasing awareness throughout our society of the devastating effects of abuse on those that have experienced it, especially in childhood. Their collaboration pre-dates the formal enquiries that churches have undergone to bring to light where their own practice has fallen short and at times has been complicit in emotional and spiritual, sexual or ritual abuse. In this, Barbara and Penny have been pioneers in their engagement, and there has at times been a sense of "going where angels fear to tread". The destructive nature of abuse, by individuals and institutions, cannot be denied, as the formal enquiries have revealed. The stories that they have heard have at times been deeply distressing, and one would like to say "unbelievable", except they are tragically true.

In the face of these horrific accounts, both Penny and Barbara have consistently been in the presence of impressively courageous women who have gone on to find strength and resilience despite the shattering of their early lives. It is true that this shattering can never be fully healed or forgotten, but there is a way of living with it and around it that does not necessarily mean defeat. This journey is often via mental disintegration, complicated relationships and lack of self-identity and worth, but it is not a hopeless journey. On the contrary, it is no coincidence that some of these women have described themselves as "freedom fighters" rather than "survivors".

Not only is this book written to share some of this learning with others; it brings reflections on how the Church could be a safer place for all people if the voices and experiences of those that have experienced trauma can critique and change the practices of an institution. It may also help those who have experienced abuse to feel less isolated by giving the opportunity to read about others' experiences. The mission of the Church has too often been based on what is said rather than how it has listened. Institutions tend to be attentive to those who speak loudest and beholden to the structures that reinforce traditional patterns of power. Yet when we give space for different stories to emerge, we not only challenge our understanding as individuals but also how we relate in every pastoral encounter, every act of worship, every church meeting and every social gathering. This is not an easy or a comfortable process, but it is an essential and ultimately life-giving one.

Words that are written on a page put a story "out there", and they also break the tyranny of oppressive people, the insistent earworms planted by perpetrators that diminish and undermine a victim. Words are powerful, and in the invitation to write, permission is given to put outside the self all those things that undermine the self. Poems and prose hold the aspirations and anguish that has so often been held in secret. They also contain a rich seam of wisdom, often unseen or unacknowledged by the author but born out of a lifetime of struggle with experiences that may have happened pre-language or never been named. This phenomenal wisdom comes from an inner voice that has sustained people through unimaginable pain. It is earthed wisdom, practical wisdom, strong wisdom, expressed by people who so often think they are worthless or have nothing to say. It is precious wisdom, transformational wisdom.

In *Writing the Wisdom*, the desire is to share some of these insights and give voice to the experiences of those who have experienced trauma and abuse. The desire also is that, through the sharing of these words and their inherent wisdom, there might be a fresh resolve in church communities to listen differently, to provide safe space for creative expression and to be open to the multi-layered narratives that are present in every place where two or three gather together. Those of us that have a faith find the wise work of the Spirit within these stories, the Spirit that was present at Pentecost enabling all people to be understood speaking in their own language (Acts 2: 1-6). Whilst we acknowledge that not everyone would choose to use the language of "God", we sense that this listening and understanding is essential to human flourishing.

And yes, this is an unfinished story; there is much more to be heard and done. Not only do all communities need to listen differently (and the Church is no exception), but they need to be open to living differently too. Whilst we have witnessed an increasing impetus to implement good safeguarding practices to enable safer spaces, we have often overlooked the stories of those who have been silenced by powerful individuals or structures. This is troubling work but also essential and transformative—this writing hopes to show, in some small way, how it might be possible.

CHAPTER 1

What are we talking about?

The word "abuse" has been much used in the media over recent times, and a number of high-profile celebrities have been shamed as abusers. Organizations such as the Football Association, the BBC, various children's homes and the Church have been named as places where abuse has been allowed to thrive. It is important that when we talk about "abuse", we don't talk in a kind of coded language and therefore in a different realm from the one we live in day to day. Whilst most people are not abusers and most people are not abused, the fact of child abuse is part of our contemporary (and historical) reality. People do hurt each other, and some children do live disrupted lives because of the actions of others. The result of these actions is trauma both in the child and in the adult abused self. This trauma fragments a person's sense of identity, their ability to form ongoing, trusting relationships and their capacity to flourish as secure and healthy human beings. This matters.

This matters, not simply because all people should benefit from the opportunities that are offered to them to live fulfilling lives, but also because we believe we are made in the image of a loving God. The fact that children are abused by adults is damaging not just to individuals but to our human communities. If one person is damaged, we are all damaged; if one person's life is fractured then we all inhabit broken communities. And if one person is able to be heard and to flourish then the whole of human society, including the Church, can grow.

When someone discloses that they have been abused during their childhood or indeed at any time in their life, it's necessary for us to listen attentively to what they're saying and feeling. They need to know that we can hear this information, that we won't deny their words and turn away. We may be the first person they've ever dared to approach, and however much they come across as attention-seeking, muddled, angry or excessively vulnerable, and however much their story may sound shocking or implausible, it is important that they don't feel disbelieved and rejected.

Whoever we are and whatever role we take within our faith community—whether we are clergy, lay leaders, pastoral visitors or members of the congregation—we are all called to be caring to those around us. If we have some awareness of the aftermath of abuse, then we are in a better position to understand and support those survivors we may encounter.

What is pastoral care?

For many Christians the term "pastoral care" may seem self-explanatory. Based on the idea that Jesus was a "good shepherd" to a "flock", the term comes out of a rural image of oversight for the church congregation, either collectively or individually. Pastoral care, therefore, is at the heart of Christian ministry, both lay and ordained; it is about offering emotional and spiritual support, being present during times of pain, praying with or for people in difficulties and a desire to see human flourishing as Jesus desired disciples to have "life in all its fullness" (John 10:10).

The image of "shepherd" is prevalent throughout the whole of the Christian scriptures, in the Psalms, the exilic prophecies of Jeremiah, Ezekiel and throughout the Gospels. The image is that of a "good shepherd" who tends and nurtures the flock with particular attention to the weakest and most vulnerable. This is a sacrificial style of leadership which embodies courage and deep care. However, if we dig more deeply into this rural ideal of pastoral attention, we can see that it also contains some challenges, not least in the power dynamics that are inherent within the imagery. Is the pastor actually responsible for church members in the same way as a shepherd is responsible for her sheep? Are the members of a congregation meek, homogeneous followers of those in pastoral oversight? Is it imperative to critique where the power lies in such an image of dependency and helplessness? And if we are looking for good practice in relation to those who have experienced trauma, is such an image of helpless dependency actually providing life-giving space for speaking out as empowered human beings? Sadly "power with" has at times been used as "power over".

Other images of pastoral care can be located within scripture. The model of "the wounded healer" is found in the Gospels in relation to the life and death of Jesus. The idea that the pastor herself is also broken, fragile and vulnerable means there can be a deep empathy in the pastoral encounter. Being a wounded carer is to stand alongside another with mutual understanding born out of a variety of life's experiences. It is not for a pastor or a counsellor to say, "I know exactly how you feel", but by our very presence and mutual understanding this can be communicated, bringing strength from weakness. The danger of such a model is that the pastor can overlook the maintenance of appropriate boundaries and, as safeguarding training teaches, it is always the responsibility of the one with power to make sure that their practice is safe.

A third model of pastoral care can best be described as "the intimate stranger". This is most often located within a chaplaincy style of ministry in which pastoral care might happen in short conversations or brief encounters. The pastor is able to have intense yet fleeting encounters with those they meet, being present to the person in the moment rather than in a formal or church setting. Jane described this model of pastoral care when she was working as a nursing auxiliary in a hospital setting, dressed in a uniform and whilst performing the most mundane tasks of patient care. She was amazed at what was confided to her simply because she was present, anonymous and had a listening ear. Often the most important and intimate confidences are shared in such brief conversations with a stranger. The danger of this model for those who have experienced abuse is that trauma often leaves someone vulnerable to trusting inappropriate or harmful people or distrustful of people with good intentions.

A preferred model for pastoral care might be that of a midwife, again a key theme of the scriptures as people are helped to be delivered from their past and find new life. The role of the hospital midwife is to accompany the expectant mother through the process of labour so that she is enabled, through unconditional care, to bring a new thing to birth. This model of pastoral care acknowledges that the pastor may be needed to be intensely present at certain times in a person's life but then to let them be independent as they nurture the new possibilities and grow. One danger of this model is that, for those who have experienced abuse, there can be inappropriate attachments and dependencies on both sides.

The last model to be explored here is the pastor as "optician"! This comes from the experience of creative writing engaged in by Penny and Barbara. The optician helps someone whose vision is blurred or out of focus by placing different lenses in front of their eyes. This starts with individual letters on a big chart and ends with a page of script. Like all analogies this image has its limitations, but it is helpful when we consider the process of creative writing. Trauma leads to the disconnection of a personal narrative, so that the experience and indeed the sense of identity become fragmented and disjointed. This can lead to a confusion of thought, an undermining of confidence and a consequent disintegration of self-worth. It is the role of the "optician-pastor" to help an individual to focus on parts of their lives that may be blurred or out of proportion. The pastor also embodies a different narrative, a meta-narrative of the creativity of the Divine. Whilst this may not be overtly referred to, it can hold the emerging story in a different light. One danger of this image for those who have experienced abuse is that the emerging story can be soaked up by the God story, so that it is diminished or not attended to properly. However, through the writing process, there can be surprising insights that produce an extraordinary weaving of words.

However we interpret the role of the pastor, as shepherd, wounded healer, intimate stranger, midwife, optician or in some other way, no model in itself is totally defining or accurate. In truth, someone with pastoral responsibilities will respond in different ways in different circumstances. What is important is to be aware of the balance of power within the pastor/pastored relationship and to maintain appropriate boundaries that always have a care for the vulnerabilities of the one who is struggling. Pastoral care is not the role of one person alone and, whilst the ordained person or pastoral visitors have particular responsibilities, they should always receive appropriate supervision and support from others.

What is counselling?

Counselling is a professional relationship between one person who is seeking help for emotional and psychological problems and another who is a trained and qualified counsellor. It is a talking therapy which enables an individual to explore their difficult feelings and experiences within a safe and confidential environment. It does not offer advice or a checklist of things to do to feel better, but rather helps uncover insight and understanding leading to greater self-awareness. Its ultimate aim is to restore hope in darkened lives and it can also bring about a better understanding of others. Some common issues addressed in counselling are addictions, bereavement, depression, relationship breakdown and trauma.

Both counsellors and pastoral carers understand the importance of confidentiality, although information should be shared if concerns are raised about the safety of any individual and especially if that person is a child.

They also respect boundaries and recognize their own limits by seeking wise guidance when they are in doubt about their own competence in coping with a situation. Every counsellor has regular monthly supervision with a more experienced practitioner in order to explore ethical issues, mistakes or concerns, and the supervisor will offer both challenge and support within a good working relationship.

There are a variety of approaches to counselling which have evolved from three main orientations: Psychoanalytic, Behavioural and Humanistic. Briefly speaking, Psychoanalysis was originated by Sigmund Freud at the end of the nineteenth century and emphasizes the exploration of the unconscious mind in order to understand all areas of the past that may be influencing present experiences. Behavioural Psychology focuses on the future achievement of new patterns of behaviour. It was developed in the 1930s from the work of Pavlov, whose research into how animals learn, which he termed "classical conditioning", brought about a whole field of studies in the ways that human beings adapt and respond to the world around them. The Humanistic approach became prominent in the 1950s and places much importance on the mutual relationship between counsellor and client. It is non-directive and concentrates on experiences in the here and now. It takes the view that each person is unique and of value, and that most people have the resources to find a way forward and discover meaning in their lives.

As the professional talking therapies have developed, attempts have been made to bring together the different ideas and methods. Many counsellors, rather than follow one particular model, prefer to combine theories and techniques from the various approaches and describe themselves as "integrative". This brings together different techniques and combines elements of particular theories to include social and political dimensions. Throughout these pages we shall be referring to a trauma-informed, integrative approach to counselling with the use of person-centred principles.

Person-centred counselling, attributed to Carl Rogers, originates from the Humanistic orientation and is centred around the three core conditions of congruence (sincere openness), unconditional positive regard (respect) and empathy, which is the ability to understand and share another person's lived experience, and which has much to do with listening to emotional truth rather than actual facts. In later life, Rogers became increasingly aware of an intuitive, mystical faculty within the use of his core conditions which links us to a reality behind the everyday world. There is a sense of something larger entering the relationship between client and counsellor, where they become vitally alive to each other. Certain changes take place. There is a feeling of joy, of trusting the present moment and of the therapist letting go of any power in order to empower the client, which in turn opens up new possibilities.

Such mutuality and care towards another is sacred and an act of spirituality.

Some religious people are wary of therapists because they are afraid that psychological ideas will disturb the basis of faith, whereas some counsellors strongly dislike certain religious attitudes and choose not to touch on spiritual matters with their clients. However, there are many people of any faith or of no religious faith at all who seek therapy in order to explore experiences which they describe as spiritual. Spirituality is difficult to define and express in words, but they speak of something that's felt as an energy presence, or a sense of oneness with the universe, or an intense affinity with nature. They might describe hearing an internal voice or word impressions. Someone who is living with the aftermath of childhood abuse may be particularly hesitant to share these things for fear of being ridiculed, or of their experiences being dismissed as "just the imagination", or even seen as a sign of serious mental disturbance. Indeed, there is a fine dividing line between the two.

One client, Megan, eventually plucked up the courage to describe an occasion when she was standing beside a lake and gazing at some trees on the opposite bank. She saw what seemed to be a brief parting in the air to reveal a much wider and outstandingly beautiful landscape, but she could find no words to describe it. Neither could she hold on to the details of what she had actually seen because it all happened so quickly. Nevertheless, she had caught a glimpse of something beyond human understanding and was left with the knowledge of a spiritual reality that lies behind our world. For Megan, it was a profoundly positive experience and one which eventually led her to the Christian faith.

The spiritual journey often reflects significant themes in a person's life and, when they are explored, it helps the person to sort through their meaning and distinguish between those things that were helpful and those that could be internalized voices from the past and therefore harmful. For many survivors, and particularly for those abused within a religious setting, God is an Almighty God who is harsh and punitive, who has power "over" rather than power "with", and who requires unquestioning obedience rather than being a loving presence who abides both within us and all around us.

Rosa, who had been brought up within a religious faith and who had been coerced into sexual activities by her father throughout childhood, wanted to know where God was at the time when the abuse was taking place. Nothing happened when she prayed; her pleas for help were ignored. Her shame ran deep because she thought that she had caused the violations and God, the male, powerful and controlling judge, knew she was bad and beyond forgiveness. She felt she had to make deals with the Almighty in order to find peace and happiness or to avert tragedy. God became the father figure who asked the impossible and then punished when that was not achieved.

Trauma and abuse

First of all, it should be acknowledged that there are many male survivors of abuse and women who abuse, but throughout this book and for the sake of clarity perpetrators will be referred to as "he" and survivors as "she", except when illustrations are given, in which case pseudonyms will be used. Individual stories are made up of a composite of experiences and any identifying details have been changed. Permission has been granted from the authors of the poems and prose writings that have been included. We use the word "survivor" to refer to someone who has experienced abuse during their lifetime, to reflect that person's courage and ability to move on and even to flourish.

Childhood abuse and neglect takes place frequently in all of society regardless of social status, race and culture and is the root cause of much criminal behaviour. It can be divided into categories of physical, emotional, psychological and sexual. Physical abuse includes injuries that have been caused wilfully and includes skull fractures, serious burns, bites, kicks and beatings. Psychological trauma is an inherent part of all kinds of maltreatment and has an ongoing negative effect on the child's psyche. Some definitions of this include: a lack of emotional responsiveness and availability, denying essential stimulation, and rejecting, devaluing or terrorizing a child. Sexual abuse is where a child is psychologically or physically forced into sexual contact such as: being made to watch sexual acts, fondled in sexual areas, forced to perform oral sex, raped or otherwise penetrated.[1] Any one of these categories would cause significant harm to an individual's spirituality. This is particularly so if there are dogmatic attitudes along with the misuse of scripture or coercive and controlling behaviour within a religious context. There is also the kind of spiritual abuse that takes place in cult groups, and we'll talk more of that later.

Over the last century and a half, awareness of sexual abuse has emerged and then been suppressed repeatedly. One example of this is when a large number of Freud's patients, who were women, revealed sexual experiences during childhood with men in their families. Initially, Sigmund Freud (1856–1939), the founder of psychoanalysis, believed that this was the cause of hysteria and called it the seduction theory, but he refused to accept that fathers abused in such a way and chose, instead, to propose that carers or more distant relatives were the perpetrators. He later renounced this idea altogether and suggested they were incestuous fantasies rather than actual events. During the 1970s, the feminist movement raised awareness and brought sexual abuse into the open along with other issues, such as rape and domestic violence.[2] In the UK, it came into the public eye during the 1980s with the Cleveland Child Abuse scandal and the setting up of Childline. More recently, the revelations regarding

Jimmy Savile and other high-profile people led to a large-scale, public enquiry into child abuse in major institutions in England and Wales.

What effects can it have?

When we experience any sort of trauma, we have to manage it, so that we do not constantly relive it. We do this in a number of different ways, and our brains help us with this process. Let's take the example of a car accident, for instance. If we have been involved in some sort of traffic accident, we will probably spend the next few weeks telling everybody about how the other driver pulled out at the junction without looking, how we tried to swerve but couldn't avoid the collision, how their anger towards us was completely unjustified. However, if we believe we were the one that caused the accident, then it may be that we are not so open about what happened. And if the accident was really serious, if we or others were injured, then it might be difficult to think about it or even remember that it happened. It might all be a bit of a blur, or maybe more of a sensation, than something we can talk about. Our brains will put the memory of the trauma away from our conscious self so that we can get on with our daily lives without having to deal with it all the time.

Abuse is traumatic, and because it often happens in childhood, it fragments who we are and how we relate to the world. Someone who has experienced abuse as a child may not have any clear memory of what has happened to them; there might be bodily sensations and pain or mysterious physical scars, but no clear narrative of events. If abuse has happened pre-speech, then it can be held in a part of self that has no words and is therefore "locked away" from the articulate adult.

The abuse may go on for years with no protection from adult caretakers. Often the perpetrator is a relative or someone in a position of trust, in which case the child is trapped beneath a veneer of respectable normality. Most young people will not tell anyone until they reach adulthood, and some never disclose it at all because they are afraid of being blamed or disbelieved. They have very likely been discouraged from speaking out or even threatened with severe punishment if they do, and so many cases go unreported.

When the trauma is ongoing and inflicted by a parent, the betrayal is particularly devastating, and in her attempts to make sense of what is happening, the child minimizes the abusive events. Added to this is the teaching from adults, both at home and at school, that parents are always right and that they always do things for her own good. She therefore believes that she is being hurt because she is different in some way, dirty, stupid or bad or all of these rolled into one. It may be too frightening for her even to consider that the fault may lie with her mum or dad and in order to maintain this all-important relationship she dissociates the abuse, locks it away in her mind and seemingly forgets about it. She then idealizes the parent and blames herself for any suffering she is experiencing. She is also likely to feel responsible for what happened if she enjoyed some of the sexual activity or the "loving" attention and gifts received during the grooming process. Self-blame allows her to retain some sense of hope and control in an otherwise helpless situation so that, if she manages to improve herself and become "good", she may one day receive the love and attention she so badly needs.[3] In the long term, however, the negative beliefs she holds about herself lead to a loss of identity alongside feelings of worthlessness, guilt and deep shame—a shame that shuts her down, shuts her out and shuts her off. Whereas guilt is about what a person has done, shame feels like inner torment and dominates an individual's life. It concerns who a person is.

Some adult survivors are more adversely affected than others and this has much to do with the age of the child when the trauma occurred, the relationship of the perpetrator, the severity of what happened and how long it continued. Some experienced very little care or protection, while others had a supportive and trusted adult who was around during the time when the maltreatment was taking place. This would make a significant difference.

Some people never forget their abuse while others have memories outside daily awareness, but which can be recalled through thoughtful reflection. Disturbing recollections might also occur when someone brings up her own child or when there is an event such as the death of the perpetrator. When overwhelming trauma occurs in childhood the memories are dissociated or pushed aside and hidden away in the unconscious mind. Dissociation is a self-protective defence, universal to all human beings, and it enables a person to separate off thoughts, feelings and events that are intensely painful, distressing or life-threatening, but it also prevents the experiences from being processed. For the one who is being abused it is as though she slips out of her body and is able to look at another, alien part of herself from a distance. This prevents her from being too overwhelmed, but over time her sense of identity is diminished and the memory of what happened becomes unreal and fragmented.[4]

Whatever the situation, there is no doubt that abuse during childhood greatly devalues people and erodes an understanding of their own abilities. It destroys any sense of hope, of inner joy, and wrecks the ability to trust. In some cases, it results in tragic consequences.

CHAPTER 2

How do stories emerge?

The healing process from childhood abuse begins when a survivor makes contact with the depths of her own story, and when this reality is acknowledged, it can be like going into battle. Life will be disrupted for a while as she wrestles to find the truth through the many years of lies—those lies she has been told by others and the ones she has told herself. It is not a linear process but cyclical, and involves the breaking down of barriers while also bringing together the fragmented inner world. It means going through the same stages many times and at different levels, but if a survivor stays with the journey and trusts its direction she will, in time, find herself moving into a much freer and more assertive way of being.

Abuse is often about power—the power of one person over another person, the power to dominate and to silence. The abuser "grooms" the victim. This means that they distort attachments to their own ends. For instance, a young child is told that Uncle X loves them more than anybody else in the world, that what Uncle X is doing is because of this love, that this relationship is their own special secret, and nobody must be told. That to tell would spoil everything; that it would lead to desperate consequences or punishment. The messages of grooming are deep-seated and hard to overrule, even in adulthood. They are "records" that play and replay, and patterns that are hard to revoke until they are recognized for what they are.

For all these reasons, it is hard for an adult who has experienced abuse to find the words. As we hear, so many people do not report abuse until a long time after the event. It is never as easy as "just saying", because the abuse survivor must first recognize what has happened to them, piecing things together from fragments of memory and sensations. They might find that these memories are held in unconscious parts of the self, and there is no sense of an integrated narrative. And because of the fragmentation of the narrative, the "story" can come out in a seemingly garbled form and is hard for others to believe.

The issue of who to tell and how to tell the experiences of the fragmented self is another layer of challenge for someone that has experienced abuse. Some first discover the story through counselling, which is often long term. Others begin to find a voice through writing. For those who want to tell their story, there is often a long process of finding the right person to tell, someone who can be trusted. There may be some trial runs to find out who might be prepared to listen—and sadly, there are many bad experiences where the selected recipient cannot or will not believe what is being told to them. This can lead to a further closing down and re-traumatization of the abuse survivor. If they are told, "Best to forgive and move on," or, "Maybe it's a false memory," or, "I'm sure it wasn't really like that," then their words are blocked once again.

Survivors are often very mindful that relating what has happened to them might also traumatize the listener. They are anxious that what they want to share might be too much to hear and upset somebody else, somebody that they respect and trust. Those of us who are called to listen have a huge responsibility to keep ourselves safe, to listen well and to find some sort of supervision that helps us to value what we have heard without suffering trauma ourselves.

Why is it hard to find the words?

Words are provisional and precious and the first steps in helping them to emerge is to believe that they are worth attending to, that they are worthy of our love and respect. The counsellor might call this "unconditional positive regard", but the Christian must see this as vocational. It is the calling of the person of faith and of the whole Church to give one another attention. This doesn't mean that we are to lay ourselves open in an un-boundaried way to the never-ending discourse of the most vocal. It means that we are called to be open to each other, to value what we hear, to be aware of our limitations and to keep confidences. This is hard work—a troubling, transformative and ultimately gospel process.

At the heart of what it means to give somebody attention is the way in which we view the "other". How many churches refer to themselves as "friendly" or "welcoming" but are in fact fearful of the outsider, or those that seemingly rock the boat? To be open to "The Other" means an openness of heart that is prepared to accept and acknowledge the uncomfortable difference of the Other, as Miroslav Volf suggests, to embrace the otherness of another and to be transformed by it.[5] To be truly open to another person means that we are prepared to be changed by them, to be part of the transformative process by which we claim our stories together. Acknowledging that in every congregation there will be the hidden stories of abuse, as there are in every gathering of humanity, means a paradigm shift. It means there is a need to acknowledge each other at much more than face value and to open up safe and boundaried spaces for stories to emerge.

What are boundaries? We need to remember that abuse is about power, the power of one person over another to their harm. People who have experienced abuse have had their boundaries violated by somebody who had power over them. It is therefore crucial, if we want words to emerge, that we are very clear about what we can do and what we can't do. To say to somebody, "I'm available any time if you want to have a chat" is probably a really unhelpful thing to do, although it feels kind. It is much better practice for us to say, "I'm sorry, I haven't got time to listen to you properly right now, but let's make a time on Thursday afternoon. I'll be free between two and three-thirty, how about we meet in Costa?" Giving clear and well-defined boundaries of time and space is crucial, as is an awareness of where there is a private space for a conversation, without it being a secret or seemingly unsafe place. And in this, we need to know our limitations. Unless we are trained as such, we are not counsellors. Giving people attention means just that, and if we find ourselves out of our depth or itching to stray beyond our levels of competence then we need to beware!

As we "listen the words into being", we need to be conscious of which promises we can keep. We may promise that the story will go no further, but if a vulnerable child or adult is at risk, then we have to talk to people. This should always be negotiated well in advance and is not a case of informing but an endeavour to keep everybody safe.

How do we make a safe space?

The honest answer to this is "We can't", as nowhere is completely safe, but we can do some things to enable a space to be safer. As indicated above, we need to be real about what we are offering, by giving people appropriate and boundaried time. We also need to be aware of our own power, even if we do not feel particularly powerful. We are powerful, and we need to use our power appropriately and only for the benefit of the person who is speaking to us. When we listen to such stories, they are precious and should not be interrupted by anecdotes of our own! If listening triggers memories for us, then we need to find somebody else to talk with.

It is always really important that people know where the exits are. These may be physical exits—leave the door ajar or ask permission to close it, always indicate that somebody isn't trapped, and always be the one that keeps an eye on the time. Or it might be emotional exits. It is probably not possible to tell a whole story in one go, so give space and have some strategies for keeping grounded. In a group setting, this creation of safe space can be constructed more overtly: the room can be set up in ways that allow for a variety of engagement and "ground rules" can be negotiated from within the group. And finally, when thinking about "safe space", it is really important that the person with the power in the conversation—the listener or group leader—has enough space within themselves to hear and engage with what is being told. We need to carry a safe space within us, an uncluttered room to welcome the guest whose words are being heard, maybe for the first time.

So we will be called to listen to people in many different ways. Sometimes we are the individual chosen by a person who has experienced abuse to hear the story for the first time. If this is the case, we need to give boundaried time and space, to honour what we hear without reproach, to understand that it might not seem to make sense and that it matters that we respond well. We may not need to be involved for a long time and we need always to be aware of our power and our limitations. On the other hand, we might be a trained listener or counsellor who is dedicated to a deep listening process, accompanying someone as they discover for themselves the reality of what has happened to them.

Whilst thinking about trauma and abuse, it is important that we stay grounded. That is, to remember that these things actually happen to real people in actual situations. However much we do not want to believe it, however much we cannot imagine how these things could happen, despite the inconsistencies and apparent gaps in stories, in the majority of cases these matters are facts, real, true experiences. If staying grounded is challenging for the one who is listening, then it can be much more challenging for the one who has experienced the abuse.

However we are asked to listen, it is a vocational and challenging activity. It calls for persistence, faithfulness and patience. Survivors of childhood abuse are in our midst. Their pain is hidden, but there's a constant, aching loneliness and a silent cry for others to dwell with them. It is not necessary to go into graphic details, but rather to take things gently, checking the person's level of emotional comfort and, as the story emerges, expressing sorrow that she has lived through such painful times. A survivor will feel supported when she's being heard in the right way, treated respectfully and given the choice to make her own decisions about a way forward.

Listening and attending—what is it and how can we do it better?

Listening is many-layered. On one level, it's something we do every day. We listen to music, to the news and other programmes on radio and TV, but how well do we listen to one another? Although we may mean well, it sometimes happens that when a person begins to talk about their troubles, we give the kind of responses that leave them feeling unheard, even rejected, and it becomes like a passing by on the other side. One example is when we offer advice and make suggestions before we've truly heard what they're attempting to say. Another is when we identify with everything they tell us by saying something like, "Oh, that happened to me . . ." and relate it to our own experience. Or we hear what's said but make a hasty judgement of the person, and either argue with them or pay little attention because we have decided that they are a bit odd or making a fuss about nothing. Then there are the times when we don't actually know how to respond or what to say and so leap into a babble of prayer with well-worn rhetoric and escape the situation altogether. There are other times when we find that something the person has said triggers a chain of private associations which bring up negative or painful emotions for ourselves and prevent us from staying with the other person's story.

Good listening validates a person and is about giving our full attention to another. It's not to stand in authority, rationalize or patronize. Rather it's to take the person seriously, laying aside our own views in order to enter into another's world with sensitivity. The one who's doing the listening doesn't interrupt or look away but tunes in and is present to the other so that together they become aware of things as they are. This kind of empathic response is to make an imaginary leap to walk in another's shoes, to see through someone else's eyes, and it is different from sympathy, where we feel sorry for someone. It's a quality that allows the other person to stand in a safe clearing where they can feel what they really feel and find an inner clarity to who they really are. It's not to change the individual, but to offer them space where change can take place, and it involves listening to the whole person—not just to their words, but also the silences that fall between the words. We hear their feelings, see their facial expressions and are sensitive to the things that are not being said or to what *is* being said, but played down. In this way, we're attending to the One who's always with us, whose presence makes our presence to each other possible, and our listening becomes a gift of healing to others.

Sometimes it helps to listen by doing something creative within a group like knitting, working with felt or clay modelling. An example of one such activity is to make a "Salt Cellar" or "Fortune Teller". These are origami shapes that many of us made in the playground at school. They involve folding the points of a square piece of paper towards the centre, turning it over and doing the same. This results in a sort of snapper into which finger and thumb of both hands can be inserted. By moving the fingers, different parts of the inside can be seen and flaps raised to reveal words or colours. In the Salt Cellar exercise, each member of the group is invited to write on one of the outside faces of the snapper some things about themselves that anyone can see, what they show to the world, what is easily known about them. This could range from "brown hair" to "cheerful". On the inner flaps are written some words about the self that are revealed to only a few people—"I'm grumpy in the morning", "I am terrified of moths"—and on the inner faces things known only to self. This is a completely private exercise and not shared with anyone else in the group, but the process is discussed. It is a helpful device in realizing how much we each keep hidden from the world and also how much others conceal their inner worlds. Knowing that others also have secrets is a help in finding the words to begin to share.

Another exercise is to write a story or experience on pieces of coloured A4 paper. This is not read out loud, but each sheet of paper is tightly rolled to form a solid tube. These tubes can then be bent or moulded to make a model that represents how the writer feels about what is written in the story. Again, the physical activity of writing and folding is helpful in finding the words.

Self-awareness

We can't give to others what we have avoided or diluted within our own lives. Sometimes we get caught up in an endless cycle of projecting our pain elsewhere or remaining trapped inside it. If we want to listen well to others, it's helpful to engage first with our own shadows—all those things about ourselves that we fear or dislike. We notice, without criticism, the complexity of our inner attitudes and how they might affect our relationships. This helps us to become self-aware and we begin to live our lives with growing sincerity, which in turn enables us to open our hearts more effectively to those who are troubled and lost. But how can we set about doing this?

One way of developing self-awareness and compassion is to keep a written journal, a very old form of self-expression in which we allow our thoughts and feelings to unravel into a notebook or something similar. Done regularly, this activity soon becomes a journey of self-discovery that enables us to move from living on the surface to going to the depths of who we really are, why we do what we do and think in the way that we think. We don't have to be particularly good at writing—correct spelling and grammar are not important—but a daily routine of allowing handwritten words to flow on to a page, like a stream of consciousness, is a transforming experience.

Focusing on something tangible, such as a stone or shell, can be an effective writing stimulus to get started. Choose one that appeals, hold it in the non-writing hand and feel it, smell it perhaps, make sounds with it if possible, even taste it. Listen to the object—not telling it what to think or say or do, but just listening and writing down whatever emerges. Our journal then becomes a private and safe place in which the masks we show to the outside world can be dropped as we let the writing guide us to where it wants to go and what it wants to be. We can reflect on our experiences and explore our imaginings, our recollections, our hopes and hidden desires through the written word.

Journal writing brings us into stillness of being and can become like a prayer or meditation that calls forth who we really are and wakes us up to areas of our life that we've avoided. Transferring our emotions in this way enables us to stand back from ourselves, clear our minds and untangle difficult or confusing thoughts and feelings. We then find it easier to let go of such things as jealousy, anger, frustration or fear, and we're able to make connections between these and how we behave and relate to those around us. It also reduces anxiety, and helps us to face and process difficult experiences and painful memories so that we can integrate them rather than let the hurts and problems control our life. Redrafting at a later date turns into a process of perceiving and understanding ourselves. It puts us on a path to movement and change. We gain insight, which in turn enables us to listen more effectively to others.

Writing—helping words to emerge

We can "tell our story", but words are never adequate to explain the whole of that reality, especially when memories are held in the body or pre-speech. Words are always a work in progress, a grasping for a language to express our identities and our experiences in this wonderful, complicated and troubling world. For people that struggle to find words, there is always an exasperating and vocational quest to choose the right combination of them, to say them well or place them carefully on the page, to work and rework the story or poem. When words do emerge, they are always like pearls of great price discovered as a shell opens just a fraction to show what's within.

Poetry and stories, both the ones we write and the ones we hear or read, have the power to awaken us to who we really are. They help us connect to one another and to the world around us. Human beings have been creating stories since ancient times, whether in drawings on cave walls or shaped in wood or through the oral tradition—stories have always been around. They are part of who we are and where we come from. They have been passed on from one generation to the next by rhythm and drums and through the written word. Whether we realize it or not we all live from within our own stories, and people read us by the things we do, the words we utter and the legacies we leave behind. To exist only at the surface of them is to be out of touch with others and ourselves. It is to be unreal.

Creativity can help us find our own unique story. Whether it is with paint or clay or pen and paper, it has the potential to open doors, reveal us to ourselves and bring us to greater self-awareness. Creative writing, when used for therapeutic purposes and wellbeing, presents us with the opportunity to make real those experiences that have never been heard previously and is a way of expressing the deepest of human emotions: sorrow, shame, love, grief, joy. It can give form to our inner world, lighten our mood or tell of the worst suffering in metaphor and storytelling. We can choose to ignore the inner, critical voices for a while, cast aside injunctions from the past that point out our spelling and grammatical mistakes, our untidiness. We can write what we need to write and then do what we like with it. It can be burnt, chucked away and forgotten about, or kept and perhaps developed at a later date. The writing of poetry and stories is a way in which we discover the ability to laugh, cry and play creatively, so often lost in the abusive childhood, and which can bring about a freedom to see things differently. It can awaken our inner being and bring us to the threshold of deep change where our sacred stories begin to rise from the dust and hold meaning that lasts.

The following chapter gives a description of how we provide intentional space for personal stories to emerge on to paper in poetry and prose, a space that enables people to play with words.

CHAPTER 3

Play with words

"Play with Words" is the name of a workshop for small groups based on listening to the self through creative writing. Its aim is to help individuals come to an understanding of their own sense of identity and intrinsic value. It is not necessary for anyone to be a poet or be able to write a gripping short story, or even to be particularly good at stringing words together, and there is no success or failure about it, no right or wrong. Neither is there any need for people to read out or show anyone what they have written, although mutual sharing along with feedback from the group can be extremely helpful and brings about a sense of connection.

Writing has the potential to put us in touch with the hidden side of our personality and may allow unfamiliar emotions and memories to emerge on to the page in words that may be surprising and seem to have come out of nowhere. Healing can begin to take place within the mutual engaging with one another's written words and in allowing that experience to bring about transformation. "Play with Words" is resourceful and self-affirming, and it enables participants to find freedom of self-expression within a safe environment. The following is a description of how one person experienced the day's workshop:

> *Heavy head and tired eyes*
> *limbs that hurt and ache.*
> *Welcome to the morning,*
> *the start of this day.*
> *When time slows down for me*
> *and chaos turns to order*
> *for a while—*
> *retreat—*
> *from life, from time,*
> *from worry.*
> *Free to do*
> *what I like to do*
> *without ridicule, criticism, cynicism*
> *or condemnation.*
> *No accusations, recriminations*
> *or illness waiting round the corner,*
> *to trap me in their world*
> *of righteous judgement—*
> *all knowing, all seeing*
> *all telling.*

"Play with Words" takes place in a room where there are no interruptions, round a table with plenty of plain and coloured paper and various writing materials. We start the day by having a few minutes of relaxation and attention to the present moment with the aim of finding some inner stillness that will enable us to see our lives with greater clarity. There are many, especially those who have experienced extreme trauma, who find this kind of "centering" exercise difficult because their minds are so restless. Nevertheless, we try to become mindful of our breathing, our inner world of thoughts and emotions, and we take time to register our senses—what we can see, hear, smell and feel in the present moment.

Out of this comes a group poem: a collective moment about being together, sharing the same space and noticing who is around us, how we feel and what we observe in the room. We write down words or phrases or whole sentences, but nothing more. We select three or four of the ones we like best and cut them into separate strips. Each one is read out, then placed on the table and the group works together to put the written strips into the order of their choosing. As a poem begins to emerge, we discover that our writing connects with others while also being personal and unique.[6]

Every participant is then invited to read an acrostic with the title of the workshop written vertically and in capitals down the left side of the page. Each line says something significant and helps to set the scene for the rest of the day, while also laying down ground rules around confidentiality and respect for one another.

Play well with the words that come to you
Listen with your ears and from your heart
Attend to others' words with kindness
You don't have to read or share if you don't wish to
Write without self-criticism
Invite the words to nourish and refresh you
Take the words gently in your hands and . . .
Hear them speak from deep places
Wise words are not necessarily complicated or difficult
Often they are simple and straightforward
Respond to the words from your feelings
Do not sprinkle them thoughtlessly, but
    let them remain confidential to us
Spelling, grammar and doing it
    right are not important.[7]

This is followed by various activities that are short and simple and help us to focus on writing creatively while also acting as a springboard for further ideas and development. An initial "warm-up" exercise is often a six-minute sprint using free-intuitive writing, an outpouring of bits and pieces all jumbled up and in no particular order. We write whatever comes and in whatever kind of language we choose. It might be unconnected words or simple phrases, scattered thoughts and impressions or passing anxieties. It involves putting down on paper anything and everything that comes and is a wonderful opportunity to blow away the cobwebs, clear the mind of clutter and free up creativity. When this piece of intuitive writing is finished, it can be put on one side until the end of the session and then read through again. Any words or phrases of interest can be marked and used to develop the writing.

A further activity might be a Haiku poem. Haiku poetry is a very short, centuries-old form of Japanese poetry that describes a distilled moment in a total of seventeen syllables divided into three lines (5–7–5). We first call to mind all the senses and then write down exactly what we perceive, describing the sights and sounds, our emotions and intuitions, just as they are in this present time:

> *A blackbird fluting*
> *in greening trees of fresh spring*
> *a world growing warm*

> *Books and toys to play*
> *paint and paper to create*
> *a space to be strong*

AlphaPoems are poems in which every line starts with the next letter of the alphabet. Childhood abuse has the power to close off spontaneous creativity, and this simple structure can act as a stepping stone towards more freedom of self-expression. It's often popular too with those who have experienced difficulties with their work in younger years. Some may have had their writing criticized or ridiculed at school and "decorated" with a teacher's red ink. They feel constrained as a result and find it helpful to work within a regular, rhythmic pattern that gives shape to their thoughts and ideas. Like most simple writing activities, the thinking process helps individuals to stay in the "now" and therefore serves as a strategy for grounding.[8]

Asking about what I find difficult to talk about
Because it's hard, frightening and worrying
Comes suddenly like a question that needs an answer
Decision
Escape
Forever avoiding
Going elsewhere and nowhere
Help my child—I try
I make a mountain out of somebody else's molehill
Jan's mountain is real, but . . .
Kindly reduced to a molehill—an unfortunate molehill
Love it
Meet it
New views
Open it
Play with it
Question it
Revisit
Sing
Talk
Understanding and patience
Visit and revisit

Welcome and question—the gift
X marks the spot—integration, whole hearted, committed
Ying and yang
Z—"In my end is my beginning"

As the process of writing unfolds, we often discover that personal material is expressed in metaphors, where we describe one thing in terms of another and shed light on those things that are difficult to access or to articulate. Turning our spiritual and emotional struggles into recognizable characters can give insight while also providing some distance from unpleasant thoughts and emotions. For example, "shame" could be reshaped into an animal, or "betrayal" could take the form of an ugly creature from another planet.[9] One survivor likened her bouts of depression to a sinister woman who often dropped by for an unwelcome visit:

> *Depression is tall and lithe. She has long bony fingers that creep their way into my darkened home—usually over a weekend. I don't know why that is. Perhaps Boredom accompanies her during her time off from the normal duties of ferrying people into the psychiatric ward. Anyway, in she comes—uninvited, shrouded in a dark purple robe while her companion Despair stands outside, tapping at the window. Depression gets very cosy. She wraps herself around me, and I really wish she wouldn't. I find her far too clingy. It takes Courage to peel her away. She doesn't like Courage, neither does she*

like such qualities as Care and Compassion. She thrives
on Loneliness. Friends are a great help. So is the pet dog.
If all else fails, I dance defiantly in the wind and driving
rain in the hope that she'll be blown away by Monday.

Another gave expression to her spiritual experience of
Wisdom. She has taken her ideas from the biblical book
of Proverbs 8:1–2. "Does not wisdom call, and does not
understanding raise her voice? On the heights, beside
the way, at the crossroads she takes her stand":

Wisdom dresses in a long, embroidered, fantastically
coloured gown with strings of patterned beads. She
stands at the crossroads like an out-of-control set of
traffic lights where red, amber and green spill into each
other, turn things inside out and become their opposites.
She's a mystery. A paradox. Most people ignore her.
Especially those in flashy cars. If they happen to glance
in her direction, they think she's far too outlandish
and way past her sell-by date. They can't see that she's
someone they've once known, but have lost touch with.
It's only those living at the edge, those who know how
to listen to her silences and wait without answers, who
understand that she's been here since the beginning,
turning stardust into gold.

The natural world often calls forth our creativity. It's
where we encounter the mysterious and a sense of our
inter-connectedness with all creation. Nature is both

magnificent and threatening. It has a calming power that inspires us with its beauty, yet also uproots us with earthquakes, storms and devastating floods. Landscapes can be full and teeming with activity or barren with little evidence of life. Mary lived for a while in an Arabian country. She described it as a remote land, dominated by mountains and with vast arid regions that stretched throughout its profoundly silent interior. She spent many days and nights camping out in the desert and began to discover her own story reflected in the landscape. She recorded her experiences in a journal and, after much redrafting, created the following:

I was fascinated by this primeval wasteland. I found the silence inviting me closer, compelling me to enter. It seeped into me, gripped me and drew me deeper into myself. I began to let go and discovered that what was out there in the shifting sands, the jagged rocks, the crumbling blistering desert—in the emptiness—was also the same as the wild wilderness of my internal world. The silence had an influence that was at times obvious, at times imperceptible, but it soon became clear that I was passing into my own symbolic desert. Fixed boundaries began to unfreeze and existing beliefs were challenged. Everything I had previously thought important wasn't important and all the things I had considered unimportant were vital. I had encountered a Love that would take me into the very depths of my being, there to face my childhood. It was only a glimpse,

*I could have pushed it away, buried it deep and for ever,
but I chose not to. I heard its silent scream, and it became
my awakening. As bad memories came tumbling forth
and hidden pain rose to the surface, there were the tears
I couldn't shed as a child, the anger I wasn't allowed to
release, the crippling shame and fears not expressed.
My early years, I realized, had been plucked away like
pulling apart the wings of a butterfly, piece by piece, so
it could no longer fly in the sunshine or feel the breeze
on its face. I was floundering and lost in a psychic storm
where everything had been reduced to chaos. It felt like
a kind of death, but this is a journey where the Spirit
hovers, where inner stillness meets outer silence—"deep
calls to deep"[10]—and in time, I found myself moving
to another drumbeat. Life became strangely different.*

Finding meaning in poetry and story

*There were three in the bed
And the little one said
No! Please Daddy, No!
Mummy let me go!*

Our parents are probably the most important people in
our lives, and the earliest interactions we have with our
mother, father or primary caregiver are crucial to our
emotional wellbeing and how we come to understand
the world around us. This is known as "attachment" and

explains how a lasting and loving bond is essential to the development of our brains in the early years of our life. In a good, secure relationship the mother is available and reliable, and she will intuitively know the needs of her offspring. She cares for her infant as if to say, "It's good to be with you. You are beautiful in every way and I adore you. No matter what happens, I will always love you for being the person that you are." The baby feels known and soothed, safe and secure, and this kind of emotional connection forms the core of his or her sense of self. It stimulates brain growth and affects the lifelong ability to engage in stable relationships. We all need to know that we are loved unconditionally, that our lives are of value and have meaning. A secure attachment tells us who we are in relation to other beings.

Adults whose attachment systems were distorted in early childhood experience problems in their later relationships. Some may find it difficult to be supportive towards their partners in times of stress, or they may fear and dismiss closeness and intimacy. Or they may be clingy and want more than their partners can provide. If a person goes on to experience new and better relationships, however, then a sense of connection to love and goodness can increase throughout life. Our early experiences of secure or insecure relationships with our parents act as a bedrock for all our future relating, including our understanding of the Divine.[11]

Here is an account of one survivor's spiritual journey that opened up painful truths about her early relationship with her mother:

When I gave my "YES" to Jesus, I meant it. I really meant it. At the time, I didn't understand that it might be a rough journey. Nobody in church told me that God has a way of probing outer defences and inner murky places that we don't know about. They talked a lot about sin though. They said that sin was the cause of all my troubles—my sadness, my addiction, my isolation. "God loves you", they insisted, but I wondered about that. What is love? Our first experience of love is our mother, the most precious of people. If we don't have that, how do we know what love really is? And where do we find it? And why was I questioning this anyway? Clearly it wasn't my problem. I'd had a perfect upbringing in a respectable family, and my parents had given me a secure and happy childhood. Nevertheless there was something there, something lurking in the deep, and I couldn't quite see it. I didn't know why this mattered. Why it felt so bad.

Then one Sunday, there were the sudden unexpected prayers in church giving thanks for our wonderful mothers, for their care and loving kindness, and ... the "something" stirred. Something unspeakable. I had a sense of being trapped in a kind of shell and realized that my life was made up of layers. My past became a constant companion as little by little, week by week, those layers peeled away to uncover painful secrets that had been hidden—even from myself. On and on it went until finally a door opened into a dark pit. A howling emptiness. A gaping wound, where trust had been destroyed and love betrayed. It was a place of no language. A place of haunting abandonment and desolation, but it was in this place that I came face to face with a part of myself I didn't know was there. A scrap of worthless humanity desperate for her mother's arms, her gaze, her safety, her love, and as I stared at this creature, the truth slowly unravelled into one long primal scream . . . and I knew with a deep knowing, that I had been emotionally neglected and sexually abused at an early age by my own mother.

My world fell apart. My infant needs came spilling out and, struggling with the emotions of a pre-verbal infant, I clutched greedily for any snippet of attention. I was desperate for someone to carry my pain and soon became attached to an older woman in a leadership position in the church who was gentle, kind and seemed to glow with maternal love. I longed for her warm smiles, her loyalty. I longed to be inwardly held and soothed as a good mother holds a wounded child.

Our relationship developed, and eventually I disclosed to her what had happened. Although I was initially heard and believed, my personal sin seemed more important than the things that had been done to me. She advised me to control all negative emotions, to forgive and move on with my life, to be lovingly

respectful towards my mother. However hard I tried,
I found it impossible to leave behind those early
childhood wounds that had determined the shape and
shades of who I had become. She quickly grew tired of
me. I was patronized, then disregarded and ignored.
Was it something I'd said? Something I'd done? Had I
been too demanding? She had been a lifeline for me, but
now a glass wall had come between us, and my dark
narrative became even darker. Overwhelmed with grief
and shame I retreated into the shadows. All I could do
was trust the thin strand of a loving Reality who was
holding me firm as I left the Church to seek the help I
needed elsewhere.[12]

Father Thomas Keating describes a process of divine therapy where our childhood wounds and unintegrated material from our early life emerges from the unconscious in a barrage of images and emotional states. He writes:

God invites us to take responsibility for being human and to open ourselves to the unconscious damage that is influencing our decisions and relationships . . . Painful memories that we have forgotten or repressed . . . Primitive emotions that we felt as children and that we have been compensating for may come to consciousness.[13]

—

In the next two poems, the writer describes her early life, where parental love and protection were largely absent. She tells the story of her experiences during childhood and, in so doing, peels away the veneer of respectability to reveal dark secrets within her family:

Normality and abuse
both living under the same roof.
An everyday scene,
unremarkable,
even serene.
What a lovely house!
What pretty flowers!
What a lovely family!
What happy, well-behaved children.
Normality and abuse,
both living under the same roof.
So ordinary, so common.
Don't look, don't listen,
shut those curtains,
shut your mind,
no horror here to find.

—

How can you grieve
without a grave?
How can you say goodbye
to one too young to die?

How can you mourn
with your insides still torn?
How can you cry
on pain meds that make you high?
A baby who died
before he knew any love.
A baby who fit
in the palm of my hand.
A baby born early,
too young to breathe.
My baby remains
buried in my mind.
No body, no ashes,
no gravestone, no sign.
Not one happy memory,
just beginning to grieve,
without even a grave.

The process of putting painful experiences down in black and white on to a page can enable those experiences to be externalized and dealt with differently. This next poem gives a clear description of how a child leaves the scene—or dissociates, in order to cope with her ordeal:

When the door closes and
darkness falls
Should I be thankful that I can't
see him,
can't see his face,

can't see the picture on it?
Is he gleeful, does he care,
does he know where I've gone,
or does he just not notice?
What's it like floating around
above the room?
No pain here, no fear.
I can see the other side of the rainbow now.
It's not as pretty,
but it forms the barriers I need.
Don't let me return to her
until he's gone please.
I know the other side of the rainbow
is grey and dull,
but oh how nice and
peaceful, safe from harm.
No one can hurt you
on the other side of the rainbow.
Only those of us like me know the way.
We just stay safe in our own cocoon
until the rainbow has gone
and the room is empty
except for her,
then we join her again
just for a while.
Maybe one day we won't have to travel
to the other side of the rainbow.
Then we can be the colours of the rainbow.
So if you see us wearing rainbow colours

please don't frown at us
Just rejoice that you've not seen
the other side of the rainbow.

Damaging patterns and cycles of behaviour dominate the lives of many children living with ongoing abuse. One woman disclosed that during her childhood her mother received regular payment for taking her to the priest's house for so-called "catechism" lessons. Another told of how her stepfather would habitually come into her bedroom early every Tuesday and Thursday morning to rape her before taking her for a swimming lesson.

Mandy described how, during her primary school years, she had been a member of the local church Sunday school. The vicar offered to take her home at the end of the afternoon class and naturally, her parents saw no reason to say "no". When Sunday school had finished and everyone had left the building, the vicar would lock the door, ceremoniously lead her up the central aisle, undress her at the altar and then proceed to rape her while simultaneously praising God with prayers and hymns. This happened once a week for most weeks and over a period of five years. Part of the grooming process had involved being told that "something went wrong when she was being made", that she had "bad blood" and that "God had told him (the vicar) to keep doing these things to her because she wasn't learning the lesson and needed to be cleansed". She was manipulated and emotionally brainwashed by repeatedly being told that these things were happening to her because she was dirty and bad and that it was all her fault.

Such a betrayal of trust is an outrage, and there is no more effective way of silencing a victim than to claim that God is sanctioning the behaviour. Mandy was nine years old when this began. She was vulnerable, alone and available, a pitifully easy target for someone in a position of power with such a well-hidden agenda and whose intentions were evil. Even if she had been able to find the right words and to pluck up the courage to articulate what was happening, who would have believed her? Her innocence had been totally plundered; she'd had little control over her life, and when she'd reached adulthood and the abuse was over, she was still controlled by the internal messages with which she'd been indoctrinated.

CHAPTER 4

What is good practice in church?

We are a community of precious, broken people. It is the responsibility of fellow Christians to listen with humility and courage—to pray, to provide protected space and offer restorative love whereby survivors can learn to reconnect with trustworthy others. Many lives have been wrecked, but they do not have to be damaged beyond repair, and it is not beyond the means of our faith communities to create a sense of belonging by engaging in life-giving patterns and rituals within a safe environment. All people need patterns that give shape to life and prevent it from descending into chaos. These patterns and rituals may be as simple as remembering to put the wheelie bin out on a Wednesday or as complicated as following a knitting pattern. These self-imposed frameworks enable us to make sense of things and to understand their true significance and meaning.

Religious organizations use these set patterns to "frame" spiritual understanding. Depending on denomination, Sunday worship may be led by a prayer book or an exuberant up-rushing of the Spirit, but whatever our faith tradition there will be a liturgical framework of some sort. This liturgical pattern reminds us of aspects of our beliefs that we might overlook so, for instance, a time of intercession is there for us to concentrate on the needs of others rather than to be totally absorbed in our own personal experience. Liturgy is not wrong, but we need to remember it is a tool for faith rather than a controller of people. Liturgy is there to empower the spiritual journey, not to enforce it. Church worship should be a safe space for us to re-centre ourselves on God and to pray for others. The experience of survivors can lead us to be mindful of some of the pitfalls that make this time less safe for everybody, and if we can learn from these experiences, we can begin to create a more open and inclusive space for spiritual exploration for everyone.

The Church as the body of Christ also has a "body language", which means that it expresses itself not only through words but in the posture it adopts in relation to the world around it. This body language signals to others whether or not it is a safe place to be, a place where you can open up safely to the many experiences of life and faith, or a place where you will be closed down. Being aware of this body language is key to the wellbeing of individuals and the whole community.

Posture and body language

Annoying though it is for any preacher when people arrive late or sit at the back of a half-empty church, thinking more closely about the body language and posture of our liturgies can begin with such a simple dilemma. For survivors particularly, it is important to be able to see and negotiate exits. This might mean sitting near the door or arriving late so as not to feel trapped. Enabling people to do this without drawing undue attention to them is really important. We must resist the desire to usher everyone into close proximity with each other, assuming that for everyone closeness means safety. Some people need space to feel safe, prefer to sit in their own corner or near the door and be in a place where they are not noticed or can escape easily.

Being asked to move around the church can also be a trigger for people who have experienced abuse. Being called out to the front can simply be embarrassing for those of us that are not born extroverts. But being asked to move to a vulnerable place can also be a trigger to bad memories. Sitting in a circle may feel more inclusive for small gatherings but, for some, to sit in a closed circle can feel like a trap, especially if asked to go into the middle to light a candle or choose an object.

Passing the Peace may involve movement or physical contact, but for those who prefer their own space, who can feel invaded or violated by the touch of a stranger, there needs to be an opt-out clause. Similarly, being asked to kneel whilst someone else, often a priest or person in control, stands over you can feel like a step too far. In these very practical ways, we can be aware of the body language of the church. If people are uncomfortable and we cannot see the reason, we may need to acknowledge that there is more to their discomfort than meets the eye. And if someone leaves the church in a rush, then there is no need to fret; it is better to resist fuss and have a named person who knows how to bring somebody out of a panic attack to go quietly and calmly to be with them.

> *I am in church on an ordinary Sunday*
> *I receive communion and return to my place*
> *it feels more appropriate to kneel there, more reverent*
> *reverence not so much for God*
> *but for the body of Christ*
> *here in this place*
> *I am struck again, as I often am at communion,*
> *by the act of this body, in this place*
> *broken*
> *And re-remembering*
> *a resurrection moment*
> *And I am there as witness*
> *as each alone and together*
> *remembers . . .*

Although considering the body language of the church might feel like a minefield, because different survivors will have very different needs, the important thing is that the church is trying to do things right, not that it always gets them right! Remembering the need for empathy and listening discussed earlier, the body language of the church needs to be open and inclusive, and this is always a work in progress. Church communities must remind themselves that for some people, just walking through the door is an act of supreme courage, and for people that have experienced trauma, those around need kind hearts, the willingness to listen, learn and hold carefully negotiated boundaries. In this respect, we are all learners.

It is also important to remember that for people who have been abused or traumatized, there is a whole back story of imposed guilt and shame. Since St Augustine reinforced conviction of sin as a starting point of faith, it has been increasingly hard for people who feel unjustifiably guilty for things for which they are not responsible to make inroads. So not only do we need to consider the body language of the church, but also the actual language that we employ. Words always convey meanings far beyond their original intention.

Guilt and shame

At the beginning of most liturgies there is a prayer of confession. Prayers of confession call to mind our sins and give us the opportunity to repent and begin again. This is really helpful if we have done something we regret or have not faced our responsibilities and is the door to returning to a right relationship with God. But if we arrive in church full of inappropriate guilt then these prayers are going to compound the issue. Putting guilt on to a victim is usually part of the grooming process, and so people who have been abused often feel responsible for what has happened. They blame themselves and feel that if they had done something differently, they would not have brought things upon themselves.

Messages are running in their head, such as "If I had been good, this wouldn't have happened to me." This sense of guilt may have been compounded by people to whom they have disclosed, if the response is something like, "Why didn't you say something at the time?" and so a feeling of shame and guilt can become a normative state, often leading to depression or other mental distress. Prayers of confession can add to this sense of guilt and shame and further alienate a person from God: "I am not good enough to be here; what if people find out who I really am?"

How is it possible to reconfigure liturgy in such a way that all the guilt doesn't land back on the ones who have least to be ashamed of? This is trickier in churches with fixed liturgies but, bearing in mind that every congregation will have at least one abuse survivor, an awareness of the inner worlds of the congregation can at least enable a different tone to words of confession, and more informal liturgies can be mindful of the need for positive affirmation of those whose level of guilt is already a hindrance to their human flourishing.

And linked to the prayers of confession is the knotty matter of forgiveness. There is usually not much of a pause between the congregation's confession of sin and the priest's absolution. A perpetrator of sin, of whatever kind, confessed in a generic way, is soon offered a path back to a loving and forgiving God. For abuse survivors, the perceived and sometimes expressed requirement for them also to forgive what has happened to them can be a huge stumbling block between them and God: "If God can forgive, shouldn't I?" And this perceived requirement can also be reinforced by messages of "forgive and forget" or "time to move on and forget the past". Often the person they need to forgive most is themselves and to be able to let go of the guilt they have no need to carry.

A general understanding of forgiveness is one that's based on repentance, truth and justice, which paves the way for reconciliation. It is not about the actual deed but about the person, and it is not a feeling but a decision. This requires the perpetrator to repent, to acknowledge openly, to take responsibility for what he has done and make sure it's not repeated. Power and control are renounced, and the result should involve a heartfelt apology and some way of putting things right. In some situations, this would involve restorative justice, which helps to repair the damage done by the offence, and which would mean a payment of some kind or even a prison sentence. Repentance opens up opportunities for the victim to be able to move on, but the value of that forgiveness is not received unless the offence is admitted. This model does not take historic abuse into account where the person has become too elderly or has died. Neither does it consider serious abuse involving the sadistic torture of babies and children. Perpetrators of this kind of trauma often have a highly manipulative pattern of behaviour where shame and blame are projected onto the victim, combined with a refusal to accept responsibility. The truth is what they fear most. They will do everything in their power to avoid the reality of the damage that they've caused.

It is important to remember that abuse is not an event in an otherwise untroubled life, but rather a disruption of self in which personal identity can become confused, interpersonal relationships dislocated and association with the world chaotic. There is no simple shortcut to forgiveness, and it certainly is not the responsibility of the abuse survivor to make it happen. If forgiveness happens at all, it will be well along the road to recovery, but if it doesn't happen then that should never be an added burden of guilt.

Language

Maybe one part of the liturgy where trauma of any kind may be acknowledged is in the prayers of intercession. Remembering to pray for people who have experienced abuse needs to be in the mind of the intercessor, and certainly more prayer resources are needed as a sensitive reminder that our vulnerabilities are not always physical and visible.

After communion in our final prayer we say
we offer "our souls and bodies to be a living sacrifice"
Many souls, many bodies
together one living sacrifice
one body.
"Sacrifice" not in terms of life given up
or demanded for restitution
but sacrifice as something made sacred
becoming holy,
becoming whole.
As the body of Christ together
we are life in all its fullness
joy and sorrow
darkness and dancing
together we hold it all.
And as I kneel, I am witness to that life, to this body:
sensing, almost imperceptibly,
as we continue this unspectacular ritual,
wholeness is becoming.

> *We share in, and witness, an act at*
>   *once both personally intimate*
> *and fully shared,*
> *we bring ourselves and our stories*
> *to this moment, here*
> *to the breaking open and the re-membering*
> *and we recognize*
> *We are the Body of Christ.*[14]

As the Body of Christ, we not only have a body language, but we have a spoken language. Church language can be quaint or full of theological jargon, but it can also be exclusive and damaging. Being aware of how we use language, how we include or alienate, brings us back to the key issues of empathy and attentiveness that we discussed earlier.

As we have discovered, in our work together as a church minister and a counsellor, words are powerful, and language has the ability to be both a positive and negative tool. In church worship, the language used is often grounded in liturgical tradition, rather than being immediate and contemporary. This gives the ability to root Christian experience in the context of history, for there to be any continuity with the past and the possibility to engage with others across the world. But language can also alienate, especially if it has been used in abusive situations to manipulate or control.

Much has been made of gender-specific references in church. The simple phrase "Loving Father God" can be for some a trigger to remember the abusive non-loving father. Bearing in mind that inappropriate attachments are often labelled as "love" for the abuse survivor, then further confusion or alienation can ensue. This is not to suggest that we totally abandon the notion of God as a loving Father, but that we are mindful of the difficulties of image and metaphor in our expression of the deity. If we only use gender-specific language, images of a God of power rather than a God who is also vulnerable, and assume the anthropomorphic nature of God over and above a non-human wisdom-based understanding, then we are limiting a relationship with God for those who find certain images difficult.

Similarly at a funeral liturgy, well-meaning clergy might want to reassure mourners that one day they will be reunited with the deceased, a source of comfort for some and terror for others. Language is a powerful tool but is always inadequate to describe the mysteries of life and death. Using a variety of descriptions and metaphors not only enables inclusion, but enriches and deepens our faith. Sometimes, however, it might be necessary to do more than simply adjust the language we use. Sometimes we need to start again and develop pastorally appropriate liturgies in response to particular pastoral situations.

New liturgies of pastoral care

We have sometimes been involved in developing new liturgies for people who have experienced abuse and who have become stuck somewhere in their relationship with God. These new liturgies are always carefully discussed and negotiated and usually involve some physical activity that enables good conversation and a safe environment in which people can express difficult truths.

One experience of such a liturgy was with somebody who had repeatedly experienced ritual abuse in a sports hut attached to a local park. Our first conversation resulted in us getting a very large piece of paper and literally throwing violent colours of paint onto it. This resulted in a mess of black and red which the individual mixed with her hands. This allowed for a great deal of anger and pain to be expressed. The painting was then left to dry in a safe space, out of sight of others who might be tempted to ask what it meant. After a further conversation, it was decided to fold the picture up into a small bundle and to take it to the sports hut. We travelled together to the venue and, after pacing around the hut and expressing more pain and hurt, the paper was burned in a drain outside the hut. We were able to say prayers and to leave something of the anguished story behind in that place.

On another occasion, someone who had experienced abuse had been to the funeral of her abuser, a member of her immediate family who had sexually abused her between the ages of three and seven. She wanted to read the passage of scripture in which Jesus takes a child and indicates that if anyone hurts them, it would be better for a millstone to be placed around their necks. This woman wrote something of her story on a piece of paper and then made a "millstone" out of clay. The paper was tied to the stone and taken to a local pond. We prayed and talked and then, with a mighty yell (and to the surprise of the ducks!), the stone and story were lobbed into the centre of the pond. This resulted in both tears and laughter but also the sense that God knew the story and there was the possibility of a different relationship with the past.

There are a number of examples of shared liturgies available, for example on the South Sydney Uniting Church website,[15] but ministers should always be aware that there are individual needs and experiences to be taken into account and that set liturgies will need to be adapted as appropriate. In doing so, it is important to keep real, to name the truth and be sure to put blame where blame is due: with the perpetrator, not the victim. Often the use of physical objects or some creative action can be helpful, but again these things need to be checked out carefully in advance, as what is helpful to one person might be a trigger to another. And liturgies should always be in the context of pastoral care. The listening, learning and compassion of the minister needs to be consistent and boundaried and with appropriate, confidential supervision. Doing it wrong can retraumatize, but getting it right can unlock the door to a new freedom, both for the one who has experienced abuse and for the wider Church.

As we have already indicated, one particular pastoral sensitivity is around the easily used word "forgiveness", a word embedded in the Church's vocabulary but often imposed as another burden of guilt on people who have experienced trauma. So we need to say at the outset that forgiveness is never a demand on the abused. It certainly does not mean a need to forget in a way that covers over the past and it is unhelpful if that is insisted upon. Painful though it is, survivors need to remember, to be angry, to put guilt where guilt is due. The act of letting go is complex. There are no straight pathways or tidy endings, and it won't happen until a survivor has lived through many levels and layers of insight and begins to understand how her past experiences have shaped the person she is becoming. It is an inner "work in progress", and may well be one that she will need to revisit repeatedly at various times throughout her life. If forgiveness is possible, then it is a mysterious gift, not another burden to add to the already overwhelming guilt instilled by perpetrators.

So we have considered the language and body language of the church and how we communicate within an inclusive and safe environment. We have seen how important it is to develop liturgies that give space for a wide variety of experiences and enable people to come as they are. We can see that our use of language is critical to the process of healing, of finding the spaces between words, of enabling stories to surface and be held alongside the story of God. This making of an "intentional space" of empathy and listening is a vocational process for the whole Church but sometimes we need to set time aside away from the business of Sundays, to allow words to flow.

We come now to the subject of "organized ritual abuse". The following chapter contains distressing material with some strong language which readers may find upsetting. It's important therefore to take good personal care whilst going through it, and it's not necessary to read it all in one go. Give yourself plenty of breathing space: for example, a walk outside to cherish the natural world or get involved with something you enjoy doing. It's also important to seek help from a trustworthy other, if required.

CHAPTER 5

Ritual abuse

There have been many reports in the media of such things as institutional abuse, sex trafficking, and organized sexual abuse in our towns and on the internet where children, and particularly girls, are being regularly exploited within grooming "rings".

Although these kinds of groups have been operating for some while and are known about these days, organized ritual abuse is only just beginning to emerge from the shadows. Michael Salter is the Scientia Associate Professor in Criminology at the University of New South Wales, Australia. He specializes in the study of organized abuse and gives the following definition:

> Ritual abuse refers to incidents of organized abuse that are structured in a ceremonial or ritualistic fashion, often incorporating religious or mythological iconography. Ritual abuse is a characteristic of particularly abusive groups and is typically associated with the torture of children and adults and the manufacture of child

abuse material. Despite vocal scepticism about the
existence of ritual abuse, it has been a feature of high-
profile sexual abuse convictions in the United States
and the United Kingdom. Professionals in a range of
contexts continue to report encountering child and
adult victims of ritual.[16]

Emma was a woman in her mid-thirties who had come
for counselling. As sessions progressed and her story
began to unfold it became evident that she had been
brought up in a family with an inverted belief system
where Christianity was turned upside down. Night-
time ceremonies of evil intent and the misuse of power,
involving the sacrifice of animals and hideous cruelty
to herself and other young children, were a regular
occurrence. It was shocking. A first reaction for many
would be one of disbelief and denial. Such atrocities
might go on in other parts of the world, but this is the
UK—a safe land of gentle rain, of birdsong and pealing
church bells. Surely, that sort of thing just doesn't
happen. Most of us would be tempted to dismiss it, to
forget all about it, but Emma's story demanded to be
heard. The secret underworld of organized ritual abuse
had opened up and our perception of humanity jolted
out of all recognition. Hers was a tale of terror, but it
was also one of creative survival.

A general understanding developed from long-term
work with Emma, and with several other clients since
that time, is that "ritual abuse" covers a broad spectrum

of group activities which often have an occult theme
to them. The group usually has an ideology which is
used to justify the abuse and the abusive rituals in turn
are used to reinforce its ideology. Regular "religious"
ceremonies take place, sometimes around specific dates
such as Halloween and the autumn/spring equinox.
The perpetrators are men and women of any age and
from all walks of life, including the priesthood. The
rituals involve repeated, extreme and sadistic torture
over an extended period of time. Amongst a variety of
sinister goings-on, young girls are splayed and shackled
to altars to be inserted with candles or crucifixes and
gang-raped. Often there is animal sacrifice and the use
of stage magic and mind control to deceive a child. Such
life-denying experiences have the power to close off
the future and, when survivors do manage to articulate
what happened to them, their stories sound bizarre and
unbelievable, which only adds to the scepticism of an
already controversial subject.

Overwhelming trauma such as this reaches its
extreme in a condition known as dissociative identity
disorder (DID), formerly known as multiple personality
disorder. DID is not something we are born with, but an
ingenious survival strategy, and is listed in the Diagnostic
and Statistical Manual of Mental Disorders, DSM-V. It
is brought about by extreme and terrifying childhood
experiences which cause the mind to fracture and divide
off into individual parts or alternative personalities
(alters). Some of these parts absorb the pain, others

observe from a distance while still others completely separate themselves off from the trauma in order to survive. Eventually these internal parts come to live separate lives with separate experiences and separate memories. They have different ages, different names and can be of a different gender, or even take a non-human form such as an animal, wizard or demon. The life story of someone with DID is full of gaps, hesitations and a set of experiences that may have considerable long-term effects such as amnesia and frequent mood changes, age regression and identity confusion. The world around her may seem unreal. She might have internal voices, feelings of possession and call herself by different names.

> *She stood.*
> *At the edge of the River of Forgetting.*
> *Not clear where the boundaries of memory ran.*
> *Where they merged.*
> *Where they meandered.*
> *The current was strong.*
> *The water murky.*
> *Too dark to see beyond.*
> *Or beneath.*
> *She saw the bridge was broken.*
> *The steppingstones were slippy.*
> *Covered in green moss.*
> *And thick, soggy algae.*
> *Hands that no one else could*
> *see held her tight.*

Trapped.
The voices moved in.

A person with this condition is not always obvious, and she will make great efforts to hide the multiplicity, but she struggles with half-forgotten childhood events that have a way of erupting quite unexpectedly into the present moment. Something prompts a memory from the past. Scenes are replayed, and the scripts retold again and again. They might occur from the sound of footsteps on the stairs or the creak of a door being opened, or it could be something as fleeting as a facial expression that reminds her of the perpetrator. An unconscious part of the mind is suddenly triggered, old wounds are ripped open and terror rises up. She may become agitated, speak rapidly and hyperventilate. Or it could be the opposite: she appears to be shut down or spaced out with a glazed look in her eyes. The person has been left suspended in past trauma-time, frozen in memories of pain and confusion which range from unpleasant emotional states to more extreme responses such as outbursts of rage, hallucinations and the sudden reliving of past events in flashbacks. These may cause her to turn to drugs or alcohol or other forms of self-destructive behaviour, such as cutting or burning, in order to deal with the emotional pain, extreme shame and sense of helplessness that she is living with. The more positive news about DID, however, is that it is possible for a person to develop co-consciousness, where the split-off personalities or dissociated parts become fully aware of one another and build good and supportive relationships. A survivor can go on to lead a creative and productive life and hold down a successful job.

When Emma first started her counselling sessions there were significant gaps in her past life that she couldn't remember. She was living with an eating disorder and a drink problem, and she self-harmed regularly to relieve some of the emotional agony she was experiencing. The path to healing called for profound courage and it was a huge risk for her to be placed at the mercy of a counsellor, to let go of hard-won control and disclose the secrets of a lifetime. As counselling progressed, her most prominent alter came forward—an angry, brave, outrageously cheeky, but loveable teenager of about fourteen years old whose name was Laura. Soon five other much younger children, all with individual names and ages, made themselves known, along with the stark memories of trauma that they held. During sessions, she would switch to a childlike part who was called "Little Girl Lost" or to another named "Leanne" and, using a rag doll to illustrate her sadistic torture, she told of the rejections, the betrayals and deceptions, the isolation of being unloved. At other times, she could find no narrative, but her story could be read in the wide, desperate eyes, the gaunt face, grey and etched with suffering. This place of shame, abandonment and raw pain . . . "My God, my God, where are you in all of this?"

The perennial question that many survivors struggle with is, "Where was God when the abuse was taking place?" Even though Emma had been told by many that God is a loving God who dwells within us and all around us and who cares for his precious children, she understandably had many doubts. In the midst of all her internal turmoil, she wrote a letter to this so-called God of Love. She poured out her desperation onto the page. She questioned, goaded, challenged and demanded answers. Then, as her trust began to grow, she invited him into her very dark and fragmented, pain-filled world.

> *Hey God!!*
>
> *I've been reading this book about a guy who met you, well, he reckoned he did. Actually, what he says is you met him. You came to Earth and spent the weekend with him. Is that true? All the words you spoke in that book about your children, about knowing and loving every single one. Do you know me, Lord? Do you love me? How come you don't come down and meet with me like you did that guy? Am I not important enough? People keep telling me that you love me with a love that I could never comprehend. I don't believe that. People tell me that I was created by you in love. Well, that's not true either is it? I can hear you inside of me now asking "What would you say if I did come down and see you face to face?" Hmmm, what would I say? Well, first of all I would ignore you! That's what I'm doing to you*

anyway, right? Ignoring you. I know for sure that you're real. So why am I ignoring you? Well, for starters, I don't understand you. And I guess also it's easier to ignore than make myself vulnerable. And the truth is, I don't believe you can help me anyway.

But then, after I ignored you for a while, I would eventually get angry with you. I would scream at you. I would scream and shout and smash things up. Hey, you're God, right? You can cope with that. But if you stay long enough, if you stick around with me, which I am not sure that you would—but if you do, you might be able to get me past the anger, to a place where I'm crying instead. You might enter with me into a place that very few people are prepared to go with me. But with you, I am able to cry, and let you see just a glimpse of the raw pain inside. And I'm not ashamed for you to see me crying. I don't need to hide my face behind anything. And as I cry, you would hold me. You would hold me tight to you. Then I would be safe—for the first time ever in my life, I would feel safe. I'm not scared to have you hold me though, as I am with others. I'm not scared. I just sit with you holding me for what seems like an eternity—and for those few minutes I feel at peace—a feeling that I long to feel. And we don't need to say anything just now, but you just know.

And then? Well, then we would talk. Slowly at first, about nothing important. And then, when you had waited long enough for me to trust you—and you would have to wait a long time for that, but if you cared enough to wait for that trust, then I would start to talk about the things that really mattered. I would tell you just exactly what it's like to be me. Down here on Earth. I hate it God. I don't want this life. Why can't you take me back with you to Heaven? Why can't I come with you? But you tell me "no", and I have to wait. I have to keep on fighting and struggling and breathing; even though every breath hurts. And I don't understand. I don't want to be here. I don't want to have the constant dilemma in my head as to whether I should live or kill myself. I don't want that choice hanging over me anymore. It's not right that I spend so many hours thinking about it. I want to die. Why would you want your child to go through so much pain? Why is this worth it? Life isn't meant to be like this.

I would tell you about how I have only just realized the truth. I thought I knew the truth before, but I was wrong. It was a false truth. And how much devastation that realization has brought me. How it physically hurts in my chest. How that pain is so great that I wish I could just lie down and die. I would tell you about how I want to run, as far away as I possibly can. But how I also know that this is something that I can't ever run from; even if I go to the other side of the world, all this will follow me. I can never outrun it and that makes me feel trapped, and scared. Whatever way I face, whatever direction I am looking, I am still trapped in this truth. It surrounds my whole being, permeates my soul. It's changed me. I am a different person now to what I was a month ago. I knew it all before, about them not loving me, about the abuse, but I didn't really believe it in my heart of hearts. Until now. The truth is, I was worth nothing. Actually I'm wrong, maybe I was worth £10. If I was lucky a bit more, but that was my worth—my worth was about how well I performed. I was born for an object of incest, of rape, an object for a group of sick perverted men to enjoy. I have even wondered these past few days if that was the very reason I came into being, the very reason I was created. I would tell you how I was beaten and neglected, how mummy couldn't even bring herself to dress or feed me, how I am not even sure that the person I called daddy was even my father. I would tell you about the deepest pain of knowing that my own mum abused me too. The greatest betrayal of them all. I was protected before, you see, denial protects you, it keeps you safe, but my safety net has been taken away. In one moment, I realized and knew and in that split second everything changed.

"Where were you? Where were you God when all that stuff was happening? Where were you?"

I scream at you now. And you say in a very quiet voice, "I was with you. I never left your side."

"Well, that's no bloody good. I didn't know that then. I was all alone then."

"But you know now," you say, "and that's enough."

"Well you know what God, that's not fucking enough. Why didn't you stop it? Why the fuck didn't you stop it?

The God of the Universe. So powerful and almighty, why the fuck didn't you intervene?"

"You know why."

And I do know why. I understand the theology shit. How you gave humans free will, but that makes no difference to me. NO FUCKING DIFFERENCE AT ALL. I don't want you to give me any theology shit. I want you to account for yourself. WHY THE FUCK DIDN'T YOU HELP ME? And you tell me that one day I will understand. Well, I am not sure that I will.

"Carry on," you say. "Tell me more."

So next, my little five-year-old steps forward. She's getting braver you see. She's more sure of herself now, and she wants to talk for herself. I am not allowed to talk for her. She tells you her name is Little Girl Lost and, like any normal five-year-old child, she trusts you. I don't know why because she's not a normal five-year-old. Never was. Never will be. And she has never trusted anyone, but she knows you are safe. She sits on your knee chattering away, and she loves the attention you're giving her. Then she starts to whisper as she tells you about the bad things. She tells you about the many times she lay awake in bed, petrified of hearing daddy's footsteps, how she would turn and face the wall and lay as flat as she could against it, almost believing that would make her disappear. She explains how if you stop breathing and hold your breath, you can hear better and concentrate more, so you can be more sure of where daddy is in the house. She tells you how she knows he is coming because she hears the doors opening and closing. She knows the different sounds each door in the house makes. The times he came into her bed and cuddled her, whispered into her ear about how special she was, "daddy's special girl". Then he raped her, day after day after day, and the pain she felt was indescribable. He did lots of other stuff too, only she doesn't know the words. She can remember it all right, she just doesn't know what to call it. She tells you how sometimes he made her do things to him too. How her hands would be really sticky from the "stuff" that came from him. How having it in her mouth nearly made her sick. She would even whisper that often she saw blood coming from herself. Then she gets scared as she tells you about the men. Those who would come to the house and pick her up with daddy, sometimes even put her in the boot of the car. You coax her on. Ask her what the men did. But she won't say anymore. A key has been locked at that point, and it hasn't been unturned yet. She can tell you about mummy though, and this is where she gets very very sad. She tells you about how mummy did bad things too. She begs you to make mummy love her. If you're God, you can do that can't you? Her little five-year-old mind has so much trust in you.

"Surely you can make mummy love me. I didn't mean to be bad. Just please make her love me." She explains to you that if you let mummy practise loving her, she might learn how to do it. If you practise something that you can't do, then in the end you are able to do it. She

will never ever understand nor accept that mummy just doesn't have the capacity to love her. She can also tell you about the beatings. How she learnt that if she rolled up into a little tiny ball against the wall then there would be less of her to kick. She will look you in the eyes and tell you that it was all her fault because she was a bad girl. How is this fair Lord? This little life should have ended right there. If you are a God who cared, this little life would have come to an end. I owe a lot to Little Girl Lost, and all my parts. They took it all for me, blocked it from my mind so I could at least try and be a normal kid. Sometimes I even think that developing DID saved my life.

Then you ask to speak to Sarah. She peeps out from her hiding place, but then goes right back to it. She won't talk to you. No way. She's hiding well away. Same as Sarah and Leanne and Immy and Mia and there are others in there hiding too. They won't speak to you. They won't come forward to even speak to the God of the Universe.

"Tell me about them," you say.

I can tell you about the day that daddy took Sarah over the path to his friends. They went into the house, and Sarah saw her daddy take the money from his friend. She understood then that Daddy had sold her. Then Sarah might whisper that she has other secrets too, that she's only just beginning to let me know about.

"If you listen to the silences," I tell you, "you might hear that which is too hard to tell. It's not what she

*does tell; it's what she doesn't or has yet to tell that's
more painful. If you can somehow listen to that which
is unspoken, then you will learn more than that which
can be told."*

*Then I tell you about Leanne. She has told us some of
the things that are unspeakable. About something called
a black mass. Your body and blood were used in her
abuse. She has told some of the absolute horrors that
happened to her, of animals being killed and blood she
had to drink. About being tied to an altar surrounded
by candles and how she gets so scared now when she
sees a candle because she doesn't understand that it's all
stopped. How she is scared that one day Satan will come
and get her, and if he doesn't, then those men will. She
will tell how she was tortured and tricked with electric
shocks. She will tell you how she hurt the baby, how she
was made to do things to another child, and she believes
that it was all her fault. I know she believes that, not
because she's told me, but because I believe it too. Can
you even come close to knowing what it feels like to
know that I was involved in a satanic cult, that I was
an object for their own wicked pleasure? Leanne knows
of the pure evil that really exists in this world. And even
though I do know a lot, I'm somehow aware that I don't
know it all. Worst thing is Lord, I didn't believe her. I
thought she was making it up. I thought it was all crap,
which must have made her feel even more alone. Maybe
she could feel that I didn't believe her, that even I wasn't
really on her side. I hope she can forgive me and learn to*

trust me. I treated her the same way everyone else did, as a liar. Turns out it wasn't lies. Turns out there really is pure evil in this world. And you God, couldn't keep that away from me. I haven't met Leanne yet. She hides from even me, only comes out when she can send me away. I want Leanne to know that I'm trying very very hard to make her feel safe. I'm trying hard to listen to her and Immy too and any others. I hope that one day they will feel safe enough to introduce themselves to me.

Then suddenly Laura jumps out. She's been listening and watching all this time, checking you out to see if she trusts you, to see if you are an ok person for us to have in our life. She pops out and tells you to "fuck off". Don't be angry with her Lord. She doesn't understand. All she understands is that we had bad things happen to us and therefore it is her job to protect us. If she feels there is a threat, then she will fight. She will fight to protect us with such a fierce protectiveness that sometimes she scares even me. You reach out to touch her hand, but she won't let you. She thinks you're gonna hurt her; she won't ever let anyone hurt us again.

"Why are you so angry Laura?" you say.

She won't tell you. She doesn't care for a God of the Universe. You mean nothing to her. Why should she care? Why should you mean anything? She also knows about the real evil that exists in this world. She knows the truth of Satan: even though he may not be a red devil with horns, she still knows that somehow he does exist. You go over to her and whisper, "It's ok. You don't need to tell me. I already know." Laura storms off. It will be a long time before she's ready to face you.

"But what would she say to me if she did?" you ask.

"You know what she would say."

"Yes I do," you reply, "but for your own sake I need you to say it."

Where do I start?

She might tell you of those binding vows where she was made to kill a rabbit to show her what would happen to her if she ever told. She made some kind of vows never to tell anyone, and even now, even all these years later, she still can't quite believe that she isn't bound by them any longer. She might tell you that she was given money to reward her for performing, that her dad was given money too. She might tell you how she was raped at knife point. She might tell you about how she knew that she had to try to always keep standing up even though they were beating her, because it's harder for them to rape you if you stay standing. But then how she had no chance in hell of being able to do that because they would beat her until she fell. She might tell you about that house by the river and being locked in that room, raped by god knows how many men, about how she was sick when they put their "things" in her mouth and made her swallow, but then the sick was wiped over her face. How even at fourteen she would pretend that she had become part of the wall, whilst she was curled up cold, naked, alone and very scared. Then how they would shower her with freezing water even in her mouth, to get rid of any evidence. Then she would stand up proud and tall and tell you how she is a brave warrior, about how she is never scared of anything, about how she will fight the battle of our life full-on because that's what brave warriors do. They fight and fight and fight and never give up. She doesn't understand that sometimes people are good or some things are healthy for me to know or that certain behaviours are negative for us. She doesn't understand that because her job is to protect, and she is so used to everything being a threat that everything to her is still a threat and she needs to protect me from that threat.

If Laura really trusts you, and I mean really really trusts you, you might just glimpse that the brave warrior is just an act, just a cover-up, a kind of protection for a very scared, vulnerable, confused teenager. A fourteen-year-old who believes she has to starve herself to keep some kind of control. A fourteen-year-old who gets so overwhelmed by her feelings that she has to cut to make sense of the pain she can't see. A fourteen-year-old who loves vodka because that makes us forget. She is a fourteen-year-old who knows about death and who is still in fear of her life. A fourteen-year-old who is even scared of being scared and has therefore made herself a brave warrior, because brave warriors are so brave, they are never scared. Then I tell you how I am so thankful for Laura because it's the brave warrior in her that I believe keeps me alive and keeps me fighting. I tell you

*how Laura is becoming my friend now, and I'm so glad
about that. She's the one who has protected us for so long.*

*So that's me. That's us. It's like I have my own little
family living inside of me, and it's hard, so hard. Living
with DID is probably the biggest challenge I will have in
my life. I wish I could say that I know and believe that
I am your child. But I don't. I wish I could say I know
how precious I am to you, but I don't.*

"*One day you will,*" *you say.*

"*I'm scared,*" *I whisper to you.*

"*I know, but perfect love casts out fear.*"

*What the fuck does that mean anyway? I can't hold
back the question anymore.*

"*When will I be free? When will you heal me?*"

"*I am healing you,*" *you say.* "*That's why I have put
you in that place where you are loved no matter what.
Where you are held and kept safe. I have given you
people to keep you safe even when you can't do it for
yourself. Can't you see that's me? And I have given you
people to journey with you, people to talk to, people to
walk with you. How can you not realize I am there in
those people?*

*How can you not see that I am there in the midst of
it all?*"

"*You know what Lord? I have so much crap in my
life, it's hard to see anything else right now.*"

*I can tell you're going now. You're getting ready to
leave me.*

"*I don't want you to go. I need you to stay with me.*"

> *You turn and smile at me. "But I'm always with you.*
> *You just have to look for me."*
>
> *Then, you're gone. And I'm alone again. All alone to*
> *deal with this shit. I don't want to do it on my own. I*
> *can't do it on my own. I hear you whisper, "Look for me."*
> *Then I get an amusing image. I can see the little baby*
> *Jesus being born in a tiny stable. And what is in a stable?*
> *Animals. And what do animals do? They shit! So, God*
> *came to earth as one of us and was born into a stable*
> *full of shit. The God of the Universe in a tiny, cold, dark*
> *stable full of shit!! I know then. I suddenly understand.*
> *My life is so full of shit, but you are able to dwell in that*
> *shit. Same as that tiny baby did 2000 years ago.*

Christ is always with us and for us, silently suffering in and through it all. Every time a fellow human being is sexually violated, emotionally and spiritually abused, Christ's hidden presence is also abused and deeply betrayed. Emma was discovering a deeper way, a trustworthy one, and although the dissociated Laura had a stubborn adolescent mind of her own, her child parts were able to share the feelings they had been secretly holding for such a long time. She was coming to understand that she had been victimized but was not a victim; she had been wounded but not destroyed and that her broken life could become a whole story.

Such stories as this raise difficult questions and hard facts that for many are too shocking to even consider. We find the land shifting from under our feet and rapidly draw a veil over what we've heard so that we can carry on as normal. Somehow we don't realize that the actions of one or a few people towards a young girl have affected all of us, and so we say "this can't be true" and banish it from our minds. Whereas we must have realistic expectations and recognize whether we're able to hear such things without being overwhelmed or even voyeuristic, it's important not to insulate ourselves against the disturbing nature of childhood abuse. Many survivors report being diminished and patronized or disbelieved and silenced, but when one member of a Christian community suffers, we all suffer. If we don't know about these things, then how can we be any kind of help to those who are struggling to survive? An attitude of being open to learn and make sense of what someone is going through will enable us to advance our understanding. We can provide a sense of belonging and offer restorative love whereby a survivor can connect with trustworthy others. When this happens, it enables her to move into a much larger world of hope and possibilities.

—

Creative writing can be a helpful tool to enable experiences of extreme trauma to be held safely and witnessed through the presence of images and metaphors that are placed within containable boundaries. AlphaPoems provide the opportunity to give voice to experiences that are difficult to articulate while also keeping them within a regular, rhythmic pattern and secure framework. The following is a courageous piece that was written by Francis, another survivor of organized ritual abuse. She was considerably older than Emma and over some years had worked through her experiences with the help of a therapist:

Am I the
Bastard who
Cuts up people and
Devours them
Eagerly
For his pleasure?
God forbid!
How can
I live under such
Judgement that links me with
His
Kind?
Let me
Never be
Overcome by this
Pleasure.
Quit my mind
Revolting Images!
Standing where I'm placed,
Unable to make a move,
Trembling inside;

Volition driven out by terror.
Whose heart is this I'm holding? His, or mine?
X-rated pictures inundate my thoughts.
Young I was then, now old;
Zig-zagging through time from now to then to now.

She wrote this next AlphaPoem a short while later and after attending the Eucharist at a cathedral. Her past torture is held by a sturdy backbone of letters from Z–A that has enabled her to give a narrative to memories of times in her life that once she wouldn't see, couldn't see or . . . dared not see.

Zealous Christian teachers filled my
Young mind
eXhortations to be good,
While in another world
Vicious perverts taught my
Unwilling hands
To do their bidding.
Spread on their altar was a child,
Replacing me; one dies, the other kills.
Quietly my soul fragments;
Panic must be buried deep inside.
Obedience is the only option given.
Nothing is certain here except more pain,
My body, soul and spirit, each in turn
Lie helpless, hopeless,
Knowing the evil of my actions.

Justice is overturned
In this place;
Hell surrounds me.
God have mercy on my soul.
Fearfully I wait my turn to
Eat forbidden flesh;
Dead now, but beating then, when
Cut by my hand from the
Body lying still before me.
Another helpless, hopeless victim.

When someone experiences this kind of trauma it brings about a feeling of being at the brink of annihilation, and in order to stay alive a human being automatically moves into a fight, flight, freeze or play-dead response. The ongoing abuse that Francis experienced during her childhood was severe, and every time it happened she desperately wanted to run to safety, but that was impossible, and neither could she fight off her abusers. Faced with this most appalling terror, her only escape was to "fly away" inwardly and observe the action from afar, as though it was happening to someone else.

The Watcher

Above the action I stand alone
Bearing witness to all I see,
Committing all my being to my task,

Daring to remember what is done;
Each word, each action.
Feeling nothing,
Guarding myself from
His power,
I remain separate, unseen.
Justice will be served if I
Keep a record of his deeds;
Looking without flinching at
Monstrous scenes,
Never turning away.
One day I will speak out;
People must face the truth.
Quiet watching is my job for now;
Rage will distract me from my task.
Suppressing all emotion, I
Train myself to watch in silence,
Understanding and remembering what I see:
Vile motivation spawning
Wicked deeds; unfolding into
eXtreme depravity.
Yet my remembering will keep her from being made a
Zero.

For reasons that we've already discussed, it's highly unlikely that a person will disclose such graphic details in a conversation at the end of a church service or in some similar situation. It's even more unlikely that she will reach out for help if she senses that others are not able to engage in any way with her story. Survivors find it difficult to respond freely to life. They are dominated by past experiences that flood the present and capture a bleak future. They often turn others away by their childish, sulky, angry or stand-offish and unsociable behaviour. If, in our faith communities, we are able to be truly human to one another and have a sincere concern for others beyond ourselves, then it's important to notice the possible signs of past trauma and/or whether it's still taking place in a person's life, whilst also recognizing when they need further assistance or professional help.

If someone seems to be attention-seeking, then before making a hasty judgement consider first whether in reality they might be care-seeking. If a person displays what seems to be an unreasonable fear of candles and crucifixes, of men in dog collars, of receiving the bread and wine or the laying on of hands, then this could be a cause for concern and should make it all the more important to offer friendship. It's not to ask probing questions or give advice; it's much more to offer the hand of mutual accompaniment and to be a faithful witness. This means hearing with the heart the dribs and drabs that a person discloses. It's about daring to stick with it and having the ability to stand firm in the midst of whatever someone needs to share. Not denying or pushing it aside, giving pious platitudes or being defensive, but staying present with a willingness to support and to offer hope.

A survivor of ritualistic abuse sometimes refers to herself as "we" rather than "I", which reflects the fragmentation she's living with. She will have lived through unimaginable terrors during childhood, often perpetrated by those closest to her, those she should have been able to rely on and trust. Depending on the nature of the group or cult, Christian concepts may have been distorted, leading her to believe that she herself is evil and unforgivable. It is extremely difficult to come to terms with these horrors and to understand how such things could possibly take place in a civilized society, but in certain given circumstances we are all capable of evil. We don't know the wounds people carry or why they do the things they do. Sometimes victims and perpetrators are one and the same person. They themselves have been emotionally abandoned during childhood and so hurt by the actions of others that they find it difficult to empathize. Their lives are focused on their own needs, and they repeat the persecution that was handed out to them. We should be careful, however, not to think that *all* those who've been violated in childhood then become perpetrators as this is both untrue and detrimental to those who are struggling to survive and rebuild their lives. If someone has been abused, it most definitely does not mean that they necessarily go on to abuse others.

As previously mentioned, a survivor is likely to blame herself for the abuse, feel responsible for what happened and to live with huge levels of guilt and shame. The first stage of recovery, therefore, is to understand that the perpetrator alone is responsible for his crime and to know that she is not to blame. The one factor present in all areas of recovery and healing is to do with "relationship", whether it's having a supportive one in childhood, a good friend or partner in adulthood or a pastoral/therapeutic one. Having a relationship also with a personal and loving God not only provides the individual with hope, but also gives meaning and purpose to life. This, along with other good relationships, help to pave the way for someone to be able to explore their thoughts and feelings, become reconciled with the excluded parts of their being and make connections between their childhood experiences and some aspects of their present behaviour.

One of the turning points towards healing is when a survivor gets in touch with her anger. Anger is disturbing, often destructive. It can roar like fire, or it can remain hidden beneath the surface simmering with jealousies, resentments and judgemental attitudes. There may be triggers that invoke internal re-enactments of the neglect and abuse that took place during childhood. Some dissociated parts will urge "attack and hit"; others will be suicidal or will say "never trust again". Still others will screech and rage with venom and revenge. There may be a dissociated part who blames the adult person for allowing the abuse to happen and that part may carry out a verbal haranguing inside the head. All of these can cause great harm to self and others, but anger also has an important message. It tells of the depth of hurt that a person's dealing with and needs to be heard. Only then is it possible for a person to move beyond explosive knee-jerk reactions or low-lying bitterness to a place where her actions become much more of an honest, steadied response. Anger, therefore, can be a catalyst for change and a sacred first step towards healing.

When a survivor embarks on the long journey of recovery, she comes to understand those parts of herself that have been acting out of childhood wounds and draws nearer to who she truly is. She finds herself travelling through a very different terrain and may be surprised by the possibilities that it brings. In time, she'll experience a benevolent spaciousness emerging between past and present and find herself able to gradually release the anger and shame, the powerlessness and the impulse for revenge while still, paradoxically, carrying her inner wounds. The pain begins to dissolve, and she becomes aware of light and colour in her life.

Deepest Amethyst

> A Myriad of colours reflect my life, sometimes they feel dark and hidden, the darkest purple, but there lies the real story, the real person, who I am, my Centre, my being.

*If you look really close, there right in the back, you will
see the precious stone; it's guarded by the layers of
colours that have served me well.
My army, my protectors, they steer off the intruders
who would love to steal the stone, or break it.
In the stillness and when it's very quiet, just sometimes
the stone comes out and, as she unfolds,
   the colours burst
forth, they dance a little and she opens up like a flower
spreading its petals.
Lilac is light and carefree; it's the part that likes to play.
Yellow and Orange are happy, they
   shine bright like a sunbeam.
Green brings life and creativity.
Silver and White are hope and peace.
Blue and Grey cast a shadow of fear and doubt; they
cling to the stone and like to surround
   it, dimming her life ...
But the deepest Amethyst is the real me, it's the life force
that gives life ...
And when no one is looking, the precious stone comes
out and dances, just for a while; and she is truly*

FREE ....

—

And Francis eventually found herself able to write the
following acrostic:

Such tenderness is in your eyes
As you gaze at my filthy nakedness.
Vile actions weigh me down with shame;
I cannot hide the guilt I feel.
Now you approach me, touch me,
God! Touching me! Not striking me dead!

Gently you start to wash me
Really clean. So gently, knowing of
All the wounds beneath the filth.
Clean at last I look into your eyes.
Enduring love flows between us.

Incarnation

The telling and writing of story is a way of grounding. As words emerge onto a page, they become a tangible and visible expression of experiences that are often only misty and mystifying. Words help us to see what is hidden, to "put it out there", to put things into a different place. Telling a story or writing a poem enables the intangible to become visible.

As a person of faith, this writing, this emergence of words can be seen to be a holy act; it is of God, part of Creation, and shows our closeness to the Creator. As we discover our own creativity, we find ourselves mysteriously close to the one who has not only created us, but all the earth. And this Creator, the maker of heaven and earth, is grounded among us in Jesus. Jesus shows us the presence of God in the real world, the here and now, this moment. God with us, incarnation, the Word made Flesh and dwelling among us.

And in the person of Jesus, the one that dwells with us and walks alongside us, we see all the trauma of what it means to be human personified. This incarnation is not about magic or happy endings or a God who acts like a Fairy Godmother, but a suffering presence entering into all the struggle and nonsense of the world. This God has a place in our own inner wisdom, shows us how we belong to everything that is created, calls us to find the goodness of ourselves.

Staying grounded is therefore a vocational activity; it is about being present to the suffering and struggles of the "other" and standing firmly yet vulnerably together in the story of God. This is not a "happy ending" sort of a faith, we don't expect God to swoop down from some heavenly realm and make everything right. On the contrary, we are committed to holding fast within the very difficult and traumatic terrain of trauma and abuse. And for the one who has suffered abuse, or continues to suffer abuse, the presence of God in the here and now, in the present moment, even in the agony of everything that is happening or remembered, is a source of hope, that despite everything all might one day be well.

Still waters run deep

Still the chaos
Still the storm
Still the anxious soul

Waters turn to Living Water
Waters turn to wine
Waters full and fine

Run down golden
Run to overflow
Run and journey on

Deep into the deep earth
Deep into silent space where
Deep calls to deep

And still waters run deep.

—

For further information about organized ritual abuse,
visit **www.firstpersonplural.org.uk**.

CHAPTER 6

Wisdom

At the raw edges of human existence, many survivors of any faith or none are aware of a guiding wisdom within themselves that is hidden yet strong and which influences the course of their healing journeys. Although there are differences in the interpretation, this source of inner guidance is a phenomenon that's consistent with long tradition, both within the major faiths and within the world of psychology and psychiatry. Psychoanalyst Carl Jung (1875–1961) acknowledged the spiritual dimension in human beings and listened to an "inner voice", both within himself and in his patients' disclosures. He talked of a source of wisdom that is deep in all of our psyches and referred to this as an archetypal image—a symbol that has gathered together many meanings and is grounded in our collective unconscious. Sigmund Freud recognized the existence of a healthy and sane part in a small corner of his patients' minds, despite the turmoil that was going on elsewhere, but didn't interpret it as being connected to anything Divine. Pierre Janet, a contemporary of Freud, who was the first to identify dissociation as a defence against traumatic events, described how one of his patients had internalized his physical appearance and the sound of his voice and when in a meditative state would ask for his advice. The answers she received proved to be far wiser and more original than anything he, Janet, could actually give.[17]

This experience of inner wisdom is called by various names, such as observing ego, higher self or internal self-helper (often shortened to ish). There are some who see it as just another dissociated part or who argue that it's caused by medication or drugs, while others say that it is unprovable and therefore irrelevant, or a fabrication in response to suggestions from the therapist. There are still others who believe it has a sixth sense and are more ready to embrace the possibility that it may have spiritual qualities, viewing it as a part of the human being that has remained untouched by trauma. In her book *Reaching for the Light*, Emilie Rose, a survivor of ritual abuse, writes:

> That tiny spark of justice within us could not be put out even in the most horrible degrading experience a human being can go through ... Every ritual abuse survivor has an inner part that somehow stayed connected to life even in the midst of torture and death ... This strong one within has a natural longing for life and healing. It is wise beyond years ...[18]

Psychiatrist Dr Ralph Allison listened to many who were living with a dissociative condition and managed to communicate with his patients' wise and higher selves. He came to the conclusion that the "ish" is inherent in every human being and is a source of healing and love, although in someone with a fragmented mind it appears to be separate.[19] These survivors are more aware of this "ish", but are unclear where it comes from. It is generally recognized as being astute, insightful and emotionally stable, offering protection to young dissociated parts and wise guidance to the adult. It can take different forms and is sometimes embellished with an image of the individual's own creation. It manifests in various ways, such as a teacher, a healer or an older self. It may include small glimmers of any kind of protective and secure figure observed during childhood, or it might be embellished with the characteristics of a safe, caring person that they've encountered at some point and which have been internalized. Sometimes clients imbibe an image of their therapist, as in the case of Janet's patient, and are able to draw on the empathy and compassion they've received throughout that relationship.

During the therapeutic process there are many conversations with dissociated "alters" that take place, but it's difficult to speak directly to an internal self-helper. It is, however, possible to collaborate in a three-way relationship between the survivor-client, the "ish" and the counsellor, and this can prove to be extremely beneficial. Brenda, who had been severely neglected and abused by her parents throughout childhood, had a self-helper called "The Sage". This was a prophet-like figure who often appeared in her dreams or imagination after particularly traumatic events. She described how this Sage would comfort and encourage her, guide her to the kitchen (often at night) and tell her where to find food and drink. When she was older and after severe self-harming episodes, the Sage would bring a sense of clarity and calm to the inner world and then help her to get to A&E, where she received medical attention.

A query arose as to how this Sage had come into existence since it had always been an adult and yet had been active in Brenda's life since early childhood. The question: "Who exactly are you?" was asked. The "ish" didn't respond directly, but later wrote in an email:

> I am not a split-off part, but I am a part of Brenda that's different to Brenda. I am what you might call a "helper". I look after her. I have no age. I don't hold specific memories and I don't take over the whole body. Instead I have responsibilities. I teach . . .

It is as though the "ish" exists on a different level with an understanding far beyond the age of the client, and there is no doubt that whatever this internal self-helper actually is, if we choose to listen with discernment it can be a resource that underpins the process of healing and provides vital support during times of crisis.

What is wisdom?

This question probably has as many answers as there are people in the world! Clearly, wisdom is different from knowledge and, although it is hard to imagine being wise if we are completely ignorant of facts, by the same token it is possible to know a lot of things but remain unwise. Wisdom is enigmatic, something that comes as a gift born out of experience rather than something that can be achieved by conscious effort. Wisdom implies a deep way of seeing that gives insight beyond the immediate events of everyday life; it can be held in the body, mind or soul. Wisdom is often born out of pain and struggle, both of individuals and of communities, even nations.

Wisdom is also deeply embedded within the spiritual life. Christian traditions talk of the wisdom of the saints, whilst the Sufi mystics bring insight and understanding from the music, songs and sayings of different sources. This is often expressed through poetry or riddle, through the sayings of wise people or the writings of the sages, but it can also be found in those who live a quieter and less noticed spiritual life. Wisdom can speak of the Divine, but it can also be ordinary and everyday.

There is also a strong theme in Hebrew and Christian scriptures in which "wisdom" is a quality used to describe a person's stature. Solomon, for instance, is described as being an exceptionally wise leader, as he could discern the will of God within human relationships. Abraham, Moses, Samuel and David were all noted for their wisdom, and this also adds to their place of honour in their leadership of the people. Abigail and Esther are less honoured, but nevertheless use their wisdom on behalf of others—we could also note here that women's stories are often underplayed in the biblical narrative and their wisdom may be described as wiliness rather than insight! In the New Testament, Mary's wisdom is honoured as she ponders her place in God's story through the words of the Magnificat, and notably others use song and poetry to express the depth of their spiritual yearning for God, in particular Anna and Simeon, who have waited a lifetime in the temple in anticipation of a messiah.

So the Bible sees wisdom as a virtue, and it has a quality that belongs to God and comes from God. Wise people are thought to be close to God; their wisdom is a gift from God and they in turn enable others to be closer to God. An understanding of this relationship has been developed most recently in the studies of many feminist theologians, who have revisited scripture to delve into the Wisdom narratives, in particular in relation to women's lost stories and experiences that have been frequently overlooked in more dominant patriarchal readings of text.

Whilst we can follow this strand of wisdom throughout biblical writings and find people described as wise, there is also another way in which the idea of wisdom is used and that is the personification of Wisdom—Wisdom is a

character who speaks and acts as if she were a person—
and yes, she is usually described as female.

In Proverbs 1:20–22 we read, "Wisdom cries out in
the street; in the squares she raises her voice. At the
busiest corner she cries out; at the entrance of the
city gates she speaks: 'How long, O simple ones, will
you love being simple?'" Wisdom personified speaks
yearningly to the people of Israel and recalls them to
their relationship with each other and with God. She
speaks in poetry and song, her voice is passionate and
often demanding, calling people back from wickedness
and showing a path for good relations and truth.

Bearing all this in mind in relation to the creative
writing, pastoral care and counselling reflected on in
this book, there have been a number of points of insight.

Firstly, keeping in mind that the wisdom narratives
within faith traditions are often expressed through
words of song and poetry, it should be no surprise that
the wisdom of the writing workshops is expressed in
literary form. The words that emerge from participants'
experiences show a depth of insight born out of
reflection on their own experiences and struggle. Words
emerge onto a page as poetry or sometimes even as
song; they are placed tentatively or sometimes flow from
somewhere deep within. Often people think they cannot
write, but with prompts or suggested poetic form, the
words invariably do appear and are always remarkable.

Secondly, whilst there was no secret that the leaders
of the group were Christians and had a personal faith,

this was never the focus for the engagement. The invitation to participants was always to express their own individual experiences through the written word, in an environment of listening and safety. They were never asked about their own faith understanding or allegiance, or even whether they believed in anything at all, and yet there were a number of very noticeable accounts of people describing the presence of "a wise one" or "overseer" or "guardian angel". These figures were particularly present in times of dissociation, and it seemed that the "wise other" had benevolent intent towards the person who was experiencing abuse. This was intriguing and began to initiate a questioning within the leaders of the group as to the place of this mysterious wisdom as a personified presence even in the darkest of times.

Thirdly, whilst the Church was at times complicit in the abuse, mostly there was a sense expressed of wisdom being a good presence or an absent presence rather than a malevolent one. The insight and language used in the participants' poetry often expressed a profound sense of "the other" and in some instances this "other" was an alter of the fragmented self, in relationship with the other parts of the self in a way that watched over the integrity of the whole person.

Fourthly, there was within the group a deep wisdom that bore witness to other participants and provided a rich seam of kindness and understanding beyond the needs of each individual. This shared wisdom went beyond the "self-help" of practical advice (although it did include this) but also accessed a larger story into which individual trauma could be placed and words discovered to express deeper truths.

The wise one—is this God?

If we return to the Wisdom literature of both the Hebrew and Christian scriptures, then there are some deep theological questions that come alongside the experiences being shared by the participants within the writing workshops. Reading the Bible with an eye to this literature gives a different narrative from that of the dominant traditional stories of the Fall, the Exodus and Christian salvation history. That is not to diminish these but rather to add another stratum to the geology of the written texts. Biblical wisdom literature provides a rich source of material, describing a poetic and mystical relationship with the Creator which honours beauty and the intensity of the human story.

In the New Testament letters to the Corinthians, we discover a reworking of an understanding of wisdom which draws us to the idea that fragility is strength: "My strength is made perfect in weakness" (2 Corinthians 12:8–10) and, counter to the dominant narrative of might being right, it also signifies a new relationship with wisdom through the resurrection: " ... but we proclaim Christ crucified, a stumbling-block to Jews and foolishness to Gentiles" (1 Corinthians 1:23). Whilst this reversal of values challenges the dominant narratives of power and strength, there are some pitfalls here for people who have been systematically groomed to feel they are worthless and silenced. Being silenced and being made to feel weak by somebody that has power over you is not what is implied by the text, and messages of "suffering in silence" are clearly not the way of God. Those who spiritually abuse others will twist texts such as these in order to make their victims compliant or silent. These are hard messages to "unlearn".

That said, it is possible to see the importance of this reversal of understanding when we listen attentively to the women in the writing group or read their poems. The stories they tell and the words they write are often presented with diffidence and fear. The grooming to which they have been subjected has systematically eroded their sense of worth and made them fearful of speech, but even though the words that actually appear on the page are often full of anguish and anger, they also frequently indicate a deeply perceptive self-knowledge and wisdom and their strength is mysteriously manifested through weakness.

Feminist theologians working with the Wisdom literature are acutely attentive to the voices that have been lost in the midst of the dominant patriarchal voices of biblical narrative. In both the Hebrew and Christian Bibles, women are often invisible or seen to be property rather than people. How true this is too of those who have experienced abuse and whose voices have been either forgotten or silenced, whose bodies have been violated and whose spirituality and emotions imprisoned. Rediscovering the theme of wisdom is to give voice to this forgotten strand of biblical understanding and insight so that those who have been overlooked can begin to tell their stories.

An understanding of wisdom also gives permission to write differently. Rather than stories having to be historically accurate or sequentially told, there is scope to write using imagery and imagination, to trawl a wide sea of language and to express profound experiences through poetry, music and art. This is a liberating process which offers the opportunity to express the deepest of confused emotions and the most fractured of stories in ways that have form and structure.

Where is God in all this?

The accounts of abuse that have emerged within the writing workshops describe times of absolute desolation, trauma, manipulation and overpowering evil. Asking the question, "Where is God in all this?" does not diminish the fact that God often seems silent, powerless and absent. Neither does "the God question" imply that God is able to fix things, will somehow magically make things all right or is expecting a denial of the traumatic effects of abuse. On the contrary, the question goes to the heart of our understanding of God's self, raising profound questions around suffering, identity and forgiveness; there is no shortcut or acceptable glib answer here.

Recognizing that no theological theory is adequate, yet wanting to honour the stories of those who have experienced abuse within the larger story of faith, presents a raft of further questions. If God is experienced as absence, then does God condone suffering? If God is experienced as present, then why doesn't God act? These questions go to the heart of the relationship of the Creator God to the person of Jesus, who God apparently allowed to suffer abandonment and crucifixion in order that resurrection could bring redemption. Here the traditional understanding of atonement for sin becomes very knotted indeed for those who have experienced abuse.

The Church has also got itself into knots about suffering and atonement, at times expecting victims to be the ones that forget their past or to be responsible for forgiving their abusers. This is to re-abuse those who have already suffered trauma and to shift responsibility away from the abuser. This damaging behaviour has often added to another layer of hurt and silencing.

Whilst it is neither possible nor the remit of this writing to unknot these theological questions, the experiences described in the writing workshops do return to the lost wisdom narratives, both of the abused and of the biblical tradition. Claiming this alternative narrative afresh does bring new understanding and hope within a spiritual journey. Together, both participants and leaders of the writing workshops have heard and learned from each other's wisdom, which has been mutually transformative and at times profoundly moving.

Wisdom, whilst enigmatic and hard to define, emerges as a mysterious gift, and when it is heard and noticed it has the possibility not simply to inform and transform a place of dark suffering, but also to transform a community. This has been experienced within the small writing workshops, and we wonder how this could go on to transform and inform the wider communities of the Church.

Often, those who have experienced abuse are not heard within church communities, as they may be considered a nuisance or a frightening presence. Stories can be diminished, suppressed or dismissed. Whilst it may not always be appropriate for traumatic stories to be shared widely or publicly, it is clear from the writing workshops that if given a safe enough space for dedicated listening, then those that have experienced trauma often have a deep wisdom that is a gift to the wider community. Rather than being "on the edge" of what it means to be church, their stories are at the heart of a God who, through Jesus, was broken and scorned, but who demonstrated what it means to claim life in all its fullness. Their wisdom can enable many to tell their stories and sing their songs.

My Saviour
I want to be dead to pain
Removed from reality, but that's not living
You came that we may live life in all its fullness
Help me to help my inner child
We look upon your risen body
Sing your praises
Speak of your sacrifice
Scars for the most part visible and spoken of.
The gaping wound in your side, the
    inner wounds hidden
Shrouded in clothing
Sanitized
Respectable.
Do you now feel your guts ripped and
    torn, the searing agony?
Let us gaze upon your brokenness
Acknowledge the unnecessary agony
Inflicted on your innocent body.
You carry all our wounds
Please let that be true.
In your brokenness we are affirmed
Understood
Accepted
Caught up in the life divine
Made whole again.

What have we learned?

We have discovered and learned a whole raft of new things. Not only the damage that is caused by trauma, particularly in early childhood, but also the astonishing strength and resilience of the human spirit. When we refer to "survivors", we are not talking about hapless victims, but many remarkable human beings who are trying to get it together despite the odds. They are making a huge journey, not to be defined by their experiences, but to make a strong claim on life's possibilities.

Recovery from childhood abuse is a long and arduous journey—a three steps forward and two steps back kind of journey. When survivors come to our retreats and writing workshops, they expect to meet others who appear damaged and different, people who reflect their own view of themselves as being inherently broken and unlovable. Instead, they encounter women who are clearly "normal" and capable, but who have gone through similar traumatic experiences. When they witness others being accepted, heard and taken seriously, they discover they are not alone. They see their own struggles of powerlessness and stigma reflected in the lives of others.

Our aim has been to offer survivors a safe place to slow down and to breathe freely, to question and reflect, to write down true feelings and thoughts and then to share with others, if appropriate. It's a time of waiting for something new to emerge and the hope is that, if possible, those who come will find the courage to break free from the suffering that is holding them in bondage. For someone to admit their shame at the feeling level in writing or in the presence of another person, or in both, is a courageous act of trust in a life where it has become so hard to trust anybody because the pain of betrayal is so deep. Here is an example of how one survivor experienced this:

> *Betrayal is invisible. It appears among people you love or friends you trust. In a moment of comfort, contentment and peace Betrayal suddenly strikes. Creeping up slowly like a mist at dawn, but with a nasty smell. Betrayal blocks out the light. You don't even think it's there until it stabs you in the back. The bleeding wound of Betrayal is hidden out of sight. What's hard to see is hard to repair. Trust has vanished in an instant, but the looming dark presence of the betrayer can't be so easily erased. The wound of Betrayal runs deep, and its friend Silence puts a surgical mask over your mouth and pushes you tight against Betrayal. No one else can see your pain, your wound or even feel the dark void that Betrayal opens in your heart. Depression falls in, sticky like black tar, to fill the hole in your heart and the wound in your back, with Emptiness taking up residence too. Ripping off the mask of Silence pushes Betrayal away, but Trust still won't return. He stays lurking just out of reach. For without him there can be no Betrayal, yet Trust feels unsafe.*

Writing within a group that is held within trustworthy and confidential boundaries is a good way of exploring personal experiences, of engaging with difficult and painful issues without trying to control them. It allows meaning to emerge from the trauma that has determined the shape of an individual's life and reflects the crossing of a threshold into unknown territory. It also bears witness to the glimpses of Something Beyond and serves as a mirror, revealing to us our own humanity. Each person's story is unique, and each piece of writing is unique; yet there is also a sense of connection and of being in communion with one another. It's a time of shared insights, of laughter and tears and of listening for all those many questions that don't have immediate answers. As Rilke wrote in his *Letters to a Young Poet*:

> Be patient toward all that is unsolved in your heart and try to love the questions themselves, like locked rooms and like books that are now written in a very foreign tongue. Do not now seek the answers, which cannot be given you because you would not be able to live them. And the point is, to live everything. Live the questions now. Perhaps you will then gradually, without noticing it, live along some distant day into the answer.[20]

There is a beauty that emerges through each person's creative writing where there is a sense of something larger. New and precious possibilities open up. When we listen and attend and journey with one another in this way, we are all changed. Wherever there is a listening heart and a relationship of mutual respect and integrity, lives touch one another, a deeper interaction takes place, one that can transform us into our truest and deepest selves.

In our work together, we have often found ourselves treading a path at the margins of both church, where many survivors can feel isolated, and the therapeutic world, where their spiritual life may be diminished or even ignored. It should be said, however, that many counsellors and psychotherapists are becoming increasingly aware of and working with their clients' spirituality in all its many shades and forms, and many church communities have developed healing and pastoral ministries that make good attempts to be supportive to the vulnerable. They are also able to recognize when a person needs other kinds of assistance or professional help and have the relevant information to hand.

However, church is somewhere that may not feel safe for many survivors. The dogma and liturgy can seem confusing and threatening with much emphasis on human sinfulness, which only serves to perpetuate their damaged sense of selfhood. For some survivors, a personal relationship with God is as frightening as the one they had with their abusers in childhood. On the one hand, Christianity teaches the importance of truth and yet on the other, sexual abuse is a secret which on no account should be revealed by the child victim. This call to truthfulness presents the survivor of organized ritual abuse with particular difficulties. A child victim may well have been threatened with death, either their own or that of a much-loved other, e.g. a pet or close relative, if they disclose their experiences. Added to this is the enforced belief that they will be doomed in the afterlife if they do not submit to the rules of the "religious" group with absolute obedience.

So what are we learning? Firstly, the need for churches, and particularly their leadership, to ask open questions, to give space and time to the complexity and difficulty of human stories that emerge. We need to implant into the mindset of church communities that not everybody's experience of life is trauma free. Indeed, it is questionable if anybody's life is as straightforward as we like to believe. Remembering that abuse is a possibility, even for people who appear to be competent and together, means that we can be more mindful of our language, of our liturgies and of our community life. This mindfulness has the potential for making life better for everyone and ultimately to transform the Church.

Secondly, we are learning that if we ask open questions, we will receive responses that may not appear to make sense. The stories people tell about their lives come from a deep place, and if there has been trauma, then this deep place may be one of brittle and broken fragments. Therefore as church communities we must learn not to dismiss people as crazy if what they are saying doesn't appear to stack up. We need to believe what we are hearing even if it doesn't seem to be factual. Whilst this is a difficult concept to grasp, mostly it means being slower to judge and more patient to listen. Stories take time to emerge; they need rehearsing and revisiting, and sometimes they need the attention of a counsellor or psychotherapist, but the first port of call is often an ordinary person with a willing ear.

And thirdly, we are learning that stories do not always emerge in a spoken way; they may be drawn or enacted. We are learning that the written word is key, especially when we let the subconscious play on paper. Permission to let stories flow in disjointed ways onto the page, to reveal the surprises that come from connecting unlikely words together, the physical activity of pencil on paper: all these offer scope for the nonsense of past experience to be seen with fresh eyes, moved into a new place and communicated differently.

We are also learning that these stories reveal profound insights into what it means to be a person of faith. It's not that people who have experienced abuse are necessarily going to be re-integrated into the Church, but rather that they have something so profound to communicate to those who have traditionally held power that the whole Church will be changed. We can no longer pretend that the Church is a flawless institution and abuses an aberration. Rather, we are all broken people, needing to listen and learn from the mistakes of the past and to be informed and re-formed in ways that allow for the complexity of the human story.

The myth of a nice God has been busted; instead we begin to glimpse the profound depth of a God in Jesus who plumbs the depth of human experience and brings light into the darkest of all places. Not a fairy-tale deity, but rather an incarnate presence, the Creator of all loving the peoples of the world back to life; the longing of God to gather the fragments of human story into the great story of redemption, to find the wide-open spaces of freedom for everyone fenced in by inhumanity.

Survivors are teaching us this. And also that life has the last laugh. The Bible reminds us that our strength is known through weakness, that the first will be last and the last first, that the poor will inherit the kingdom of God. Survivors are not called to sort out the Church, rather they have a prophetic call to the Church to listen and learn. Their stories may be horrendous, but those who tell them are not. These fragile, vulnerable, strong people have insights into the presence of God that will call the Church and the world to account. We ignore them at our peril!

But if we do listen, then there is the possibility, by God's grace, for a painful redemption and a new vision of what we could all become as we write a different story together.

Reflection

In the end . . .
when my eyes have dimmed and
this journey's through,
can I say that
I've lived my life
in truth?
Can I say that
I've entered a gate
to the sacred, engaged
with the divine,
explored my own darkness and
reclaimed the shadows—
those feared and rejected parts?

In the end . . .
when I'm bent with age and
this journey's through,
can I say that
I've opened my heart to
the silenced, the betrayed,
the frightened and lost?
And will I have listened
and heard
and known
and lived into
God's loving response . . .
In the end?[21]

Useful organizations

The Survivors Trust: **www.thesurvivorstrust.org.**

National Association of People Abused in
Childhood (NAPAC): **napac.org.uk.**

Notes

1   J. Briere, *Child Abuse Trauma: Theory and Treatment of the Lasting Effects* (London: Sage Publications, 1992).

2   J. L. Herman, *Trauma and Recovery* (London: Pandora edition, 2001).

3   F. de Zulueta, *Trauma and Attachment: Developmental Trauma in Adults: A Response to Bessel Van der Kolk* (London: Karnac Books Ltd., 2008).

4   <https://www.firstpersonplural.org.uk/>, accessed 3 November 2021.

5   M. Volf, *Exclusion and Embrace: A Theological Exploration of Identity, Otherness, and Reconciliation* (Nashville, TN: Abingdon Press, 1996).

6   C. Moskowitz, "Group Poem: The making of a group", in G. Bolton, V. Field, K. Thompson (eds), *Writing Works: A Resource Handbook for Therapeutic Writing Workshops and Activities* (London: Jessica Kingsley Publishers, 2006), pp. 51–2

7   A debt to the former Orchard Foundation (Bristol, UK) that's informed this work.

8   G. Bolton, V. Field, K. Thompson (eds), *Writing Works: A Resource Handbook for Therapeutic Writing Workshops and Activities* (London: Jessica Kingsley Publishers, 2006).

9   R. J. Gendler, *The Book of Qualities* (New York: Harper & Row, 1988).

10 Psalm 42:7.

11   J. Bowlby, *Attachment and Loss Vol.1: Attachment* (New York: Basic Books, 1969/1982).

12   First published in "Reflect and Respond", <https://www.methodist. org.uk/safeguarding/support-for-survivors/survivor-resources/>, accessed 3 November 2021, © Trustees for Methodist Church Purposes, 2020.

13   T. Keating, *The Human Condition* (Mahwah, NJ: Paulist Press, 1999), pp. 24–5.

14   Face2Face Lent Conversations: <http://holyroodhouse.org.uk/face2face>, accessed 3 November 2021.

15   <http://www.southsydneyuniting.org.au/liturgies/2013/november-3. html>, accessed 3 November 2021.

16   See <https://www.organisedabuse.com/>, accessed 3 November 2021.

17   C. Comstock, "The Inner Self-Helper and Concepts of Inner Guidance: Historical Antecedents, its Role within Dissociation, and Clinical Utilization" *Dissociation* 4:3 (1991), pp. 165–77.

18   Cited in A. Miller, *Healing the Unimaginable* (London: Karnac Books Ltd, 1996).

19   R. Allison, *Minds in Many Pieces: Revealing the Spiritual Side of Multiple Personality Disorder* (Los Angeles, CA: CIE Publishing, 1999).

20   R. M. Rilke, *Letters to a Young Poet*, quoted at <https://www.goodreads. com/quotes/717-be-patient-toward-all-that-is-unsolved-in-your-heart>, accessed 3 November 2021.

21   First published in "Thresholds", <http://www.bacp.co.uk>.

EU GPSR Authorized Representative:

LOGOS EUROPE, 9 rue Nicolas Poussin, 17000 La Rochelle, France

contact@logoseurope.eu

www.ingramcontent.com/pod-product-compliance
Lightning Source LLC
Chambersburg PA
CBHW070405200326
41518CB00011B/2076